# GENETIC
# RESPONSIBILITY

# GENETIC
# RESPONSIBILITY

## On Choosing Our Children's Genes

### Edited by

## Mack Lipkin, Jr. and Peter T. Rowley

*Departments of Medicine, Psychiatry, and Pediatrics*
*and Division of Genetics*
*The University of Rochester*
*School of Medicine and Dentistry*
*Rochester, New York*

**PLENUM PRESS • NEW YORK AND LONDON**

154930

301.243
G-328

Library of Congress Cataloging in Publication Data

Main entry under title:

Genetic responsibility.

    Proceedings of the symposium "Genetics, Man, and Society," held at the American Association for the Advancement of Science meeting, Dec. 29, 1972, and sponsored by the Task Force on Genetics and Reproduction at Yale University and the Youth Council of the American Association for the Advancement of Science.
    Includes bibliographies.
    1. Genetic engineering—Social aspects—Congresses. 2. Medical genetics—Congresses. 3. Genetic counseling—Congresses. I. Lipkin, Mack, ed. II. Rowley, Peter T., ed. III. Task Force on Genetics and Reproduction at Yale University. IV. American Association for the Advancement of Science. Youth Council. V. Title: Genetics, man, and society. [DNLM: 1. Genetic counseling—Congresses. 2. Genetics—Congresses. QH431 G3282 1972]
QH442.G46                    301.24'3                  74-12149
ISBN 0-306-30813-4

Proceedings of the symposium "Genetics, Man, and Society,"
held at the American Association for the Advancement of
Science Meeting, December 29, 1972

© 1974 Plenum Press, New York
A Division of Plenum Publishing Corporation
227 West 17th Street, New York, N.Y. 10011

United Kingdom edition published by Plenum Press, London
A Division of Plenum Publishing Company, Ltd.
4a Lower John Street, London W1R 3PD, England

Printed in the United States of America

# FOREWORD

The "Genetics, Man, and Society" symposium was a collaborative effort of the Task Force on Genetics and Reproduction at Yale University and the Youth Council of the American Association for the Advancement of Science (A.A.A.S.). The Task Force on Genetics and Reproduction at Yale is a voluntary, inter-professional organization engaged in examination of ethical and social implications of medical and basic genetics. It is similar in purpose to the Hastings Institute of Society, Ethics, and Life Sciences and the Kennedy Center for the Study of Bioethics at Georgetown. The Youth Council of A.A.A.S. was a committee of the A.A.A.S. concerned with problems of young persons. The Youth Council had significant impact on the A.A.A.S. through the constitutional reform and a number of innovative programs including the Congressional Fellows and Regional Centers Program, and the Committees on Minorities and Women. The symposium was initially conceived by William Drayton and Richard A. Tropp and was arranged by us. The Task Force took primary responsibility for format and for selecting and inviting speakers. The Youth Council made the arrangements, raised the necessary funds and represented the organizers for post-symposium use of the materials including printed and taped publications. This volume contains the edited proceedings of the symposium plus the editors' perspective on it.

The structure of the volume reflects the conviction of the organizers that new genetic knowledge uncovers problems whose solution must include an entire spectrum of perspectives. Rational decision-making in genetics requires knowledge of the available scientific facts, personal and psychological insight, the perspective of society from social scientific and moral viewpoints, and a sense of the social mechanisms available and their limitations. Thus the volume begins with what is known about human genetics and progresses to discuss the implications of this new knowledge.

The symposium was made possible by generous grants from the following foundations:

The *National Institute for General Medical Sciences* of the National Institutes of Health of the Department of Health, Education, and Welfare under grant number NIH 73-C419.

The *Joseph P. Kennedy, Jr.* Foundation, Washington, D.C.

The *Commonwealth* Foundation, New York.

The *E.R. Squibb & Sons, Inc.* Foundation, Princeton, New Jersey.

The *Russell Sage* Foundation, New York.

Funds were administered through the American Association for the Advancement of Science by Dr. Richard Scribner.

Mr. Ronald Williams, Dr. Richard Scribner; the four panel coordinators, Dr. Maurice J. Mahoney, Ruth Silverberg, Reverend Richard Van Wely, and Richard A. Tropp; and the Youth Council Committee of David Burmaster, William Drayton and Harold J. Raveche, each made invaluable contributions to the quality of the day. We remain most grateful for their help.

Mack Lipkin, Jr., M.D.
Rochester, New York

David C. Duncombe, Ph.D.
New Haven, Connecticut

# CONTENTS

## IV.  HOW CAN SOCIETY'S DECISION-MAKING INSTITUTIONS BE MADE TO FACE THE LONG-TERM CONSEQUENCES OF INDIVIDUAL GENETIC CHOICES?

## V.  EDITORS' PERSPECTIVE

## VI.  SUGGESTIONS FOR FURTHER READING

# INTRODUCTION

The symposium "Genetics, Man and Society" deserves publication for several reasons. The papers and discussions can initiate the general reader to the current level of debate concerning genetic issues. We desire thus to stimulate the collection of more and better data, the construction of more formally acceptable philosophy, and the design of better defined strategies of change. The widest possible public debate of the issues raised by the panelists is paramount.

As editors, we have tried to increase clarity and enhance coherence. We have asked authors to respond to the opposing views of other panelists. We have added a concluding essay that draws a few lessons from the symposium and urges collection of the data most needed to add an empirical basis to the theories and attitudes of genetic decision-makers.

We are most grateful to Dr. Hugh Cline and the Russell Sage Foundation for a generous grant to cover costs of editing. Roberta Ferron, Lynda Wood and Patricia Horton have been indispensable to the preparation of the manuscript and we thank them. It has been a pleasure to work with Johnson D. Hay and John S. May of the *Daily Record* and Phyllis Straw of Plenum Press.

We especially thank each author for accepting painful mutations in the manuscripts.

We thank Lawrence E. Young, Robert J. Haggerty, Philip L. Townes, Richard A. Doherty, George L. Engel, Sanford Meyerowitz, and Arthur H. Schmale for stimulation and support.

Mack Lipkin, Jr., M.D.

Peter T. Rowley, M.D.

*Editors*

*Rochester, New York*

May 17, 1974

# I. PROGRESS AND PROBLEMS IN MEDICAL GENETICS

# MEDICAL GENETICS:
## PROGRESS AND PROBLEMS

### Leon E. Rosenberg, M.D.

*Professor and Chairman, Department of Human Genetics,
Yale University School of Medicine, New Haven, Connecticut*

It is entirely fitting that the Youth Council of the A.A.A.S. should select the field of medical genetics for a symposium. I say this because medical genetics is a youthful field, conceived in this century, infantile until a mere quarter century ago, and currently undergoing a most dramatic adolescent growth spurt. In fact, the field has many of the emotional characteristics of an adolescent — boundless energy and optimism coupled with impatience and a modicum of naivete. In my remarks, I shall take my cue from the ebullient spirit of this young field and attempt to convey the sense of excitement and challenge which those of us engaged in the study of medical genetics feel today.

## BIOLOGICAL PERSPECTIVE

Each human cell contains enough DNA to code for about seven million proteins.[1] If, as has been suggested, only 10 percent of this DNA is functionally active, this still provides a complement of approximately 700,000 proteins to regulate and modify human growth, development and homeostasis. Since only about 1 percent of these proteins have been identified chemically or genetically, the function of the vast bulk of man's genetic machinery remains to be elucidated.[2]

This genetic material is constantly changing. Based on current estimates of the rate of human mutations and the number of genetic loci coding for proteins, the total number of mutations expected *per* germ cell is between 5 and 10.[1] Most of these mutations are clinically neutral — that is they cause no overt disease — but their continuing presence emphasizes the great potential of such mutational events in the etiology of the numerous inherited metabolic or chromosomal disorders known or yet to be discovered.

We are only beginning to appreciate the magnitude of overt disease produced by genetic or congenital abnormalities. Approximately 5/1000 newborns in the U.S. suffer from major chromosomal abnormalities with lethal or substantial clinical consequences.[3] In addition nearly 2000 different, identified phenotypes result from single gene effects inherited in classical Mendelian manner — these mutations are responsible for clinical abnormalities in perhaps 10/1000 newborns.[2] About half of these mutant phenotypes are inherited as autosomal dominant traits; this means that they are detectable when the mutation has altered only one of the pair of genes, or alleles, at any given autosomal locus. An additional 40 percent are inherited as autosomal recessive traits and are observed in individuals homozygous for the mutant gene, implying that the mutation has altered both of the alleles at the involved autosomal locus. The remaining ten percent of mutant phenotypes are sex-linked, meaning that the mutation has occurred on the X, or sex, chromosome. In the United States alone, it has been estimated that more than 20,000 children are born per year with major chromosomal or biochemical disturbances. These congenital disorders rank second only to malignancy as causes for mortality in children under 5 years of age and may be responsible for as much as 50 percent of all pediatric hospital bed occupancy.[4] An even larger group of individuals develop disorders such as diabetes, high blood pressure and schizophrenia in which less well defined genetic factors play an important causative role.


## RAPID PROGRESS

In my introduction I said that the field of medical genetics is characterized by rapid progress. Let me illustrate with a few examples. The entire discipline of medical cytogenetics, the study of normal and abnormal human chromosomes, has evolved during the lifetime of everyone older than eighteen. It was only in 1956, a mere 18 years ago, that cytogeneticists learned that each human cell contains 46 chromosomes — 22 pairs of autosomes and 1 pair of sex chromosomes. Three years later Down's syndrome was shown to be due to the presence of a single extra chromosome. In the ensuing decade many other disorders were described whose manifestations could be traced to the presence of too much or too little chromosomal material or to rearrangements of this chromosome complement. In the past two years newer staining techniques have been described which now permit accurate identification of each different human chromosome and this technologic advance is already being translated into descriptions of previously unrecognized disorders and clarification of known conditions which could not be completely understood by older, less specific methods of chromosomal identification.[5]

The discipline of human biochemical genetics is older — 72 years old to be exact — but is still a product of our century, largely of the past 30 years. It is only 25 years since sickle cell anemia was shown to be due to a structural abnormality in the hemoglobin molecule and only 20 years since phenylketonuria was traced to a specific deficiency of the enzyme, phenylalanine hydroxylase. We now know of more than 100 different human diseases caused by specific abnormalities of a single protein.[6] Some of these diseases like hemophilia or thalassemia result from inherited disorders of proteins which circulate in the blood. Many others like muscular dystrophy, cystic fibrosis and Tay-Sachs disease are caused by mutations which affect intracellular enzymes in the liver, brain, kidney and other solid tissues. New biochemical diseases are being described at an exponential rate and these descriptions go beyond simply identifying the particular protein or enzyme involved to the more complicated questions of how these proteins become abnormal and how single protein abnormalities lead to a great range of clinical consequences.

Even more recent are advances which are currently drawing together the fields of chromosome structure and gene function. The ability to propagate human cells in tissue culture and to fuse such cultured cells with other mammalian cells — either human or non-human — has permitted investigators to begin to localize specific genes to specific chromosomes.[7] The human gene map is still only rudimentary. But more progress in mapping the human autosomes has been made in the past three years than in the preceding thirty and this endeavor is truly just beginning.

## DISEASE MANIFESTATIONS

Genetic disorders produce a huge array of clinical consequences which differ enormously in type, severity and age of onset. For instance, some chromosomal anomalies interfere with fetal development so profoundly that they lead to spontaneous abortions in the first trimester of pregnancy. Other chromosomal rearrangements produce minimal overt physical change and are compatible with long and normal life. Similarly, metabolic disorders, which lead to internal biochemical dysfunction rather than gross anatomic disturbance, may damage the fetus, be lethal to the newborn, produce symptoms only in adulthood, or even be totally harmless. Where a particular disorder falls on this broad spectrum depends on the nature of the function subserved by the particular gene locus involved and on the degree of functional impairment produced. Thus, partial deficiency of a vital enzyme may kill, while complete deficiency of a non-vital one may go unnoticed unless specifically assayed.

## DIAGNOSTIC APPROACHES

There is nothing unique about the medical methods used to establish the diagnosis of an inherited disease: historical information, physical signs, chemical abnormalities, x-ray changes. What is unique is the way these tools are used to extend the information on one patient to the family or even to society. It is the predictive and preventive power of genetics which I want to emphasize with two examples.

Phenylketonuria (PKU) is a disorder of amino acid metabolism in which the amino acid phenylalanine accumulates in blood and urine because its breakdown is blocked by a specific enzyme defect (in phenylalanine hydroxylase). This disturbance leads to severe mental retardation, and, in the past, most patients with this disorder spent their lives in institutions. In the past decade this dismal picture has been improved significantly for three reasons. First, knowledge of the inheritance pattern of PKU now allows parents of an affected child to know that each pregnancy carries with it a 25% risk for recurrence. Second, the disorder can be detected by a simple blood test in the first days of life. Third, it has been established that a diet restricted in phenylalanine can prevent the mental retardation. In this instance, prenatal diagnosis can both prevent delayed disease manifestations and allow parents to make intelligent decisions about future pregnancies.

Down's syndrome (or as it is unfortunately called, mongolism) also produces mental retardation but for a very different reason. In this condition, each cell contains 47 chromosomes rather than 46. In some unexplained way, this extra chromosomal material causes the characteristic facial features and mental subnormality characteristic of this illness. Down's syndrome is easy to diagnose but responds to no known treatment. Therefore, regardless of how early in life the diagnosis is made, the prognosis for the affected patient is the same. In this instance, the recently achieved ability to propagate human cells in tissue culture has changed the clinical impact of the disease. For, as you shall hear from Dr. Kaback subsequently, it is now possible to culture fetal cells—obtained by withdrawing a sample of amniotic fluid—and hence make a diagnosis of Down's syndrome early enough in pregnancy to permit therapeutic abortion if that is the family's desire. Here, the geneticist has focused the diagnostic searchlight on the unborn rather than the newborn, because it is the only possible site at which intervention can eliminate the human cost and burden of a disease.*

## THERAPY

It is apparent from my previous remarks that, in the case of PKU, diagnosis goes hand in hand with treatment whereas this is not the case for Down's syndrome. This difference between metabolic and chromosomal disorders exists for many other conditions. To my knowledge, no definitive therapy for any chromosomal abnormality exists or is on the horizon. However, an increasing variety of therapeutic tools are proving to be effective in preventing the sequellae of *metabolic* disorders. Like PKU, several conditions respond to dietary restriction of a substance which cannot be metabolized normally. In other disorders whose manifestations result, not from accumulation of a compound, but from deficiency of a product, either oral or parenteral replacement of the product may circumvent the mutation and restore normal or near normal function. In still other disorders characterized by a partially blocked enzymatic reaction, administration of drugs or specific vitamins may stimulate enzymatic activity enough to overcome metabolic dysfunction.[6] None of these approaches attempts to replace the defective protein or enzyme, but this, too, is feasible in several instances. If the protein normally circulates in the blood, then replacement should be relatively simple, as exemplified by the use of anti-hemophilic globulin in the treatment of hemophilia.† Tissue protein replacement presents a much more formidable task, but there is at least one possible example now of effective enzyme replacement brought about by organ transplantation. In the disorder of lipid metabolism called Fabry's disease, renal transplantation has resulted in a marked biochemical and clinical improvement. Apparently transplantation provides the mutant host with a new source of an enzyme deficient in his own tissues.[8] This very exciting, recent development must be watched closely, for, if it is accompanied by long-term success, it will undoubtedly find use in many other related diseases for which no effective therapy is currently available.

---

*Much can be done, of course, to make the best of the birth of a child with Down's syndrome. Here and below, Dr. Rosenberg is referring to treatment of the genetic defect and its biochemical and anatomic effects and not excluding the possibility of significant supportive treatment of affected persons—Eds.

†Although replacement of a circulating protein is conceptually simple, practical replacement therapy requires instruction in intravenous administration and costs of materials may be, in hemophilia, as high as $18,000 per year — Eds.

## PROBLEMS

But enough of the progress. What of the problems? No field which has grown so rapidly could be without them, and medical genetics has problems aplenty: problems in the continuing exploration of the molecular nature of chromosome structure and enzyme function; problems in understanding the mechanisms by which chromosomal or biochemical lesions produce overt or covert clinical illness; problems in delivering the fruits of genetic research to the sick people who need them; problems in educating physicians about the principles and practice of this field of medical genetics which has escaped many doctors because it has been developing too rapidly and too late for them to have assimilated its essentials; problems in informing the public honestly as to what they can expect from this field, and, perhaps more importantly, what they cannot expect; and, last but certainly not least, problems in convincing the executive branch of our government that continuing progress in medical genetics depends on adequate financial resources for the training of new professionals in this field and for the support of laboratory and clinical investigations so crucial to future human gains.

## CONCLUDING REMARKS

I shall restrain myself from discussing such potential progress and problems as in vitro fertilization, directed mutation, and selected viral transduction for two reasons. First, because some of these topics will be discussed subsequently. Second, and more important, because I believe that such discussions are, in the main, premature at this time. I believe that the diagnostic and therapeutic methods in current use — such as amniocentesis, heterozygote detection, genetic counseling, life long diet or drug treatment, and organ transplantation — present us today with so many formidable medical, social and ethical questions that it is unnecessary to grapple, yet, with the societal issues of scientific approaches so distantly, if even perceptibly, on the horizon.

## References

1. NEEL, J.V. Thoughts on the future of human genetics. *Med. Clin. N. Am.*, 53: 1001-1011, 1969.

2. McKUSICK, V.A. *Mendelian Inheritance in Man. Catalog of Autosomal Dominant, Autosomal Recessive and X-linked Phenotypes*, 3rd edition, Baltimore, Johns Hopkins Press, 1971.

3. LUBS, H.A. and RUDDLE, F.H. Chromosomal abnormalities in the human population: Estimation of rates based on New Haven newborn study. *Science, 169:* 495-497, 1970.

4. ROBERTS, D.F., CHAVEZ, J., and COURT, S.D.M. The genetic component in child mortality. *Arch. Dis. Child., 45:* 33-38, 1970.

5. CASPERSSON, T., ZECH, L., JOHANSSON, C., and MODEST, E.J. Identification of human chromosomes by DNA-binding fluorescing agents. *Chromosoma, 30:*215-227, 1970.

6. ROSENBERG, L.E. Inborn errors of metabolism In *Diseases of Metabolism*, 7th edition (P.K. Bondy and L.E. Rosenberg, editors), Philadelphia, Saunders Publishing Company, 1974.

7. RUDDLE, F.H. Linkage analysis using somatic cell hybrids. *Adv. Hum. Gen., 3:* 173-237, 1972.

8. DESNICK, R.J., BERNLOHR, R.W., SIMMONS, R.L., NAJARIAN, J.S., SHARP, H.L. and KRIVIT, W. Enzyme therapy for Fabry's disease. *Program and Abstracts, The American Society of Human Genetics*, p. 23a, 1972 (abstract).

# GENETIC EVALUATION OF THE HUMAN FETUS IN UTERO: PRESENT AND FUTURE PERSPECTIVES

Michael M. Kaback, M.D.

*Associate Professor of Pediatrics and Medicine, Associate Chief, Division of Medical Genetics, Harbor General Hospital, UCLA School of Medicine, Torrance, California*

Rapid progress is being made in the science of human genetics. Methods developed primarily in microbial systems for the detailed study of genes and their actions, can now, in some instances, be extended to the study of man. These scientific accomplishments, coupled with changing social and legal attitudes, provide important and challenging new tools for the physician-geneticist.

One immediate focus for these technical innovations concerns the application of recently gained knowledge to the genetic evaluation of the human fetus early in gestation. A simple and relatively safe obstetrical technique — trans-abdominal amniocentesis — can be utilized as early as the 12th to 14th week of pregnancy to obtain a sample of amniotic fluid from the uterus of a pregnant woman. Cells of fetal origin are present in this fluid and with techniques of somatic cell cultivation they can be grown in the laboratory. From these dividing cultures of amniotic fluid cells, an accurate determination of the chromosomal constitution of the fetus can be made within a few weeks after amniocentesis. Many genetic-metabolic parameters of the fetus can be assessed in these cultured fetal cells as well.[1] Since many serious and currently untreatable genetic disorders are associated either with aberrant chromosomal constitution or with specific biochemical abnormalities (inborn enzymatic deficiencies), such conditions can be identified in the midtrimester fetus in this fashion. Table I lists those conditions which have been detected successfully in the second trimester fetus with these methods.

With widespread changes in societal attitudes toward abortion, life quality, and population control, these technical capabilities provide important new alternatives for many families. A couple, at a defined and predictable risk for a serious inherited disorder in their offspring, can now be provided a mechanism by which they can have their own children without

**TABLE I: GENETIC-METABOLIC DISORDERS DETECTED ANTENATALLY IN THE MIDTRIMESTER HUMAN FETUS**

| DISORDER | ABNORMALITY IN AMNIOTIC FLUID CELLS |
|---|---|
| Chromosomal aberrations (Down's syndrome, etc.) | Abnormal karyotype |
| Fabry's disease | Deficient $\alpha$ galactosidase activity |
| Galactosemia | Deficient gal-l-P uridyl transferase activity |
| Gaucher's disease | Deficient glucocerebrosidase activity |
| Glycogen storage disease, Type II (Pompe's disease) | Deficient $\alpha$ 1, 4-glucosidase activity |
| GM$_1$ gangliosidosis, Type I (generalized gangliosidosis) | Total acid $\beta$ galactosidase deficiency |
| Hunter's syndrome (MPS II) | Abnormal kinetics of $^{35}SO_4$ incorporation |
| Hurler's syndrome (MPS I) | Abnormal kinetics of $^{35}SO_4$ incorporation |
| Krabbe's disease (globoid leukodystrophy) | Deficient cerebroside-$\beta$ galactosidase activity |
| Lesch-Nyhan syndrome | Deficient hypoxanthine incorporation, deficient HGPRTase activity |
| Lysosomal acid phosphatase deficiency | Deficient acid phosphatase activity |
| Maple syrup urine disease | Deficient branched-chain keto acid decarboxylase activity |
| Metachromatic leukodystrophy | Deficient arylsulfatase A activity |
| Methylmalonic aciduria | Deficient methylmalonylCoA isomerase activity |
| Neimann-Pick disease | Deficient sphingomyelinase activity |
| Tay-Sachs disease | Deficient hexosaminidase A activity |

fearing the birth of such a seriously afflicted child. This can be achieved through intrauterine monitoring of the fetus with each pregnancy. Where genetic studies show the fetus to be unaffected, the pregnancy may continue without further anxiety. Where the fetal cell studies show the fetus to be affected, the family, once informed, can elect to terminate (abort) the pregnancy if they so choose. In this way, many families, who in the past might have been fearful of even attempting a pregnancy because of genetic disease in a close family member or in a previous offspring, now can be aided to have unaffected children selectively.

In certain instances, an increased risk for a specific genetic abnormality may be known to exist **not** because of a previous affected family member, but rather because of certain demographic, ethnic, or religious characteristics of the family. Pregnancies in women of advanced reproductive age have been associated with a dramatically increased risk for offspring with significant chromosomal abnormalities. Sickle cell anemia occurs most in descendants of black Africans. Tay-Sachs disease occurs in infants of jewish parents with Central or Eastern European ancestry (Ashkenazi). These are but a few samples. With further application of recently developed "screening" techniques, it may be possible to identify individuals and couples at-risk for such disorders from within the high-risk subpopulations even before a first affected child is born. If intrauterine fetal monitoring for the condition is available, the at-risk couple so identified could be helped to have only unaffected offspring. Certain prototype programs of this type have been initiated already.[2] The intrauterine diagnostic capability provides the "positive" reproductive alternative upon which such screening programs have been developed.

As improved techniques become available for screening healthy individuals for the carrier state of deleterious recessive genes (and thereby for the potential of serious genetic disease in their progeny), extension of existing preventive programs is likely. It must be emphasized that the thrust of such programs should be to prevent the tragic impact of serious untreatable genetic disease and not to manipulate or "engineer" the genetic constitution of any population. In addition, the necessity for informed consent and voluntary participation in such genetic screening efforts, with full recognition and respect for differences in individual attitudes and beliefs, must be maintained in such efforts.

Although a substantial number of serious genetic disorders can be detected in the fetus through amniotic fluid cell analysis, a much larger group of inherited diseases cannot be identified as yet in this way. Certain heritable conditions with major structural abnormalities in the fetus (e.g., absence of brain, failure of closure of the spinal canal) are not regularly associated with chromosomal or known biochemical abnormalities. In addition other diseases are not reflected in amniotic fluid cells and might be detected only in specific tissues (e.g., blood). These problems might be resolved if a safe and reliable method for direct visualization of the fetus were available. Serious structural abnormalities in the fetus could be directly observed or samples of blood or tissue might be safely obtained if the site for sampling could be carefully and safely chosen. A number of laboratories in the U.S. and other countries are currently developing such fetal visualization and tissue-blood sampling instruments.[3] It is anticipated that within the next few years safe and reliable instruments for these purposes will be available.

Radiologic and related techniques might be used for assessing fetal structure but distinct limitations and potential hazards exist with each of these approaches. With a visualization-sampling capability a large number of serious disorders could be accurately detected in early fetal life.[4] But here, as with "routine" amniocentesis, a potential for "misuse" must be considered. How does one define "serious, untreatable, genetic disease"? Will fetal evaluation for the purpose of selecting the sex of one's offspring be acceptable? How much and to what degree will such technological tools foster an intolerance for "imperfection" in our society? Such questions are vital to the advancing frontiers of fetal medicine.

It is important to emphasize that detection of genetic disease in the fetus need not relate only to potential abortion. It may be possible in the not-too-distant future to consider initiation of effective therapies for certain genetic disorders during fetal life. In this manner the expression of the abnormal genetic condition might be offset. With continued research into the early diagnosis of genetic disease and into the basic pathogenetic mechanisms involved, it is likely that techniques for intrauterine fetal therapy will evolve.

Further investigation into the physiology of the uterus during pregnancy and the control of premature labor could permit, as in several animal species, direct surgical procedures on the human fetus. This would allow for anatomical correction or treatment of serious fetal defects of either genetic or nongenetic nature.

The technology for genetic evaluation of the human fetus has developed rapidly in recent years. Further developments are very much anticipated. The applications of this technology may be of great benefit to individuals, families, and to society at large. A potential for misapplication, however, also exists. It is essential therefore, that careful and wise consideration be given these new tools if both man and society are to benefit from such innovations.*

*Supported in part by grants from the National Foundation March of Dimes and the President's Fund — California Institute of Technology.

## References

1.  MILUNSKY, A., LITTLEFIELD, J.W., KANFER, J.N., KOLODNY, E.H., SHIH, V.E., and ATKINS, L. Prenatal genetic diagnosis, *New Eng. J. Med.* 283: 1370, 1441, 1498, 1970.

2.  KABACK, M.M., ZEIGER, R.S. Heterozygote detection in Tay-Sachs disease: A prototype community screening program for the prevention of recessive genetic disorders, *Adv. Exp. Med. Biol.*, 19:613, 1972.

3.  VALENTI, C. Endoamnioscopy and fetal biopsy: A new technique. *Am. J. Obstet. Gynecol.* 114:561, 1972.

4.  KAZAZIAN, H.H., KABACK, M.M., WOODHEAD, A.P., LEONARD, C.O., NERSESIAN, W.S. Further studies on the antenatal detection of sickle cell anemia and other hemoglobinopathes. *Adv. Exp. Med. and Biol.* 28:337, 1972.

# IN VITRO FERTILIZATION AND ITS USES IN ANIMALS AND MAN

Benjamin G. Brackett, D.V.M., Ph.D.

*Associate Research Professor and Managing Director of the Primate Colony, Department of Obstetrics and Gynecology, Division of Reproductive Biology, School of Medicine, and Department of Animal Biology, School of Veterinary Medicine, University of Pennsylvania, Philadelphia, Pennsylvania*

## INTRODUCTION

Fertilization is the process in which spermatozoon and ovum come together and unite to form a zygote. Initially, the sperm cell penetrates through the surrounding cellular investments, the zona pellucida, and into the vitellus of the ovum. Fertilization proceeds as the sperm head enlarges to form the male pronucleus and, following activation of the ovum, the female chromatin condenses to form the female pronucleus. Ovum activation denotes the resumption of meiosis which proceeds from metaphase II to completion. Male and female pronuclei develop and come into apposition, pronuclear membranes break down, and the chromosomes from male and female gametes intermix. Mitosis begins and fertilization is concluded with the first mitotic metaphase which is rapidly followed by cleavage into a two-cell embryo. Fertilization takes approximately 12 hours in the rabbit and roughly twice that in large domestic animals including (wo)man.

Fertilization has been accomplished outside the body, extracorporeally or in vitro, for several mammalian species (see Brackett, 1973 for review).[1] These include the cat,[2] gerbil,[3] guinea pig,[4] hamster,[5] man,[6] mouse,[7] rabbit,[8] rat,[9] and squirrel monkey.[10] Studies of in vitro fertilization are important in leading to a better understanding of gamete union. Most of our knowledge in this area has evolved during the last quarter of a century. Efforts have been largely directed toward defining physical and chemical conditions that allow fertilization to take place outside the body. These efforts are still underway.

## DOCUMENTATION FOR THE OCCURRENCE OF FERTILIZATION IN VITRO

The most convincing criterion of successful in vitro fertilization is the birth of young resulting from ova inseminated and cultured to early cleavage, then transplanted into foster mothers. In this way, M. C. Chang in 1959, first demonstrated that ova of a mammalian species, the rabbit, could be fertilized in vitro and proceed to develop into live young of both sexes.[11] Ovum cleavage has been widely used as a criterion for the occurrence of fertilization. The reliability of this criterion is questionable until the experimental system has been proven to result in authentic fertilization by additional criteria. Cleavage of ova resulting from degeneration or from parthenogenetic activation must be ruled out before cleavage alone can be equated with completion of fertilization. A valuable control (no-sperm control) involves ova which are manipulated in exactly the same way as inseminated ova but with no exposure to sperm cells. When no cleavage occurs in such a control, the insemination step can be concluded to invoke the changes resulting in cleavage.

Documentation for the occurrence of fertilization in vitro should show involvement of the sperm cell in the process. Male offspring resulting from transfer of in vitro fertilized ova and demonstration of the Y chromosome introduced into the ovum by the sperm cell are means of satisfying this requirement. Sperm penetration and sequential development of fertilization can be directly observed and filmed by time-lapse cinematography. Extracorporeal fertilization has been documented in this way in the rabbit[12] and in the hamster,[13] and such documentation provides convincing evidence of the sort needed to support claims of human in vitro fertilization. Sperm involvement can also be followed by examination of ova at varying intervals after insemination.

## IN VITRO FERTILIZATION AS AN EXPERIMENTAL TOOL

In vitro fertilization provides a useful tool for morphological and biochemical studies of sperm penetration of ova, of polyspermy, and of other abnormalities of fertilization. Application of presently available knowledge should facilitate continued testing of the ability of sperm populations to fertilize ova under widely varying experimental conditions, including alterations in medium or surrounding atmosphere, addition of chemical substances, or experimental treatment of ova, spermatozoa, or both prior to insemination. It should be possible, eventually, to acquire sufficient knowledge of the fertilization process to enable scientists to develop means by which gamete union might be enhanced or inhibited in a controllable way. Such means might be useful in treatment of infertility or in contraception. The value of such knowledge is apparent in light of the population explosion, the desire of people to limit their family size, and the need to limit certain animal populations for reasons of public health and economics. On the other hand, enabling people who wish to have children to be able to do so, and enhancing the reproductive efficiency both of livestock and of endangered species to prevent their extinction all provide ample motivation for research in this area.

## IN VITRO FERTILIZATION AS A PRACTICABLE PROCEDURE

Direct application of extracorporeal fertilization procedures can be predicted to receive widespread human and veterinary clinical usage in the future. However, at the present time, procedures involving in vitro fertilization are not developed sufficiently for clinical usage. Clinical application of extracorporeal fertilization as a means of circumventing blocked oviducts in human patients may be predicted. But much more extensive animal experimentation is a desirable prerequisite of such efforts in humans. Answers to questions concerning the risks involved, along with the anticipated incidence of success, must first come from animal experimentation. The most successful experiments along these lines have been accomplished with rabbits[14] and mice.[15] In rabbits and mice, only about 10% probability can presently be predicted for success in obtaining an ovum from an ovarian follicle, carrying out in vitro fertilization, and obtaining a live offspring after surgical transfer of the resulting embryo into the female reproductive tract of a surrogate dam. Additional experiments, carried out in rabbits to support the potential for future clinical application of this procedure,[16] confirm the low probability of success for any single ovum, whether recovered from an ovarian follicle or following ovulation from the ovarian surface. Beginning with an in vitro fertilized rabbit ovum that has been cultured to the 4-cell stage, the probability of its development to term following transfer is less than 20% based on our most recent data. The surviving offspring are apparently normal and when mature they are capable of normal reproduction. The present low incidence of success in rabbit studies and the dearth of experience with other animals provide insufficient encouragement for immediate, direct clinical application of these procedures to human patients.

To this day, no one has been able to achieve extracorporeal fertilization with gametes of large domestic species. Nevertheless, future application of in vitro fertilization should be expected to receive greatest impetus in efforts to improve livestock production since such efforts are exempt from many ethical considerations involved in the treatment of human patients. A consistent procedure by which cow ova could be fertilized in vitro would be of value in combining gametes from animals with desirable genetic traits. Resulting embryos could be transferred into female reproductive tracts of less valuable (but not less fertile) cows for development into desirable calves. Further development of methods of embryo transfer and for storage of ova will augment the usefulness of a repeatable procedure for extracorporeal fertilization. Another direct practicable application of in vitro fertilization would be for facilitation of early testing of the ability of bull sperm to penetrate ova after frozen storage of the sperm. This application might allow early elimination from artificial insemination programs of bulls that yield sperm which cannot be successfully stored.

## NEED FOR ADDITIONAL BASIC RESEARCH

Prerequisites for the development of a practicable procedure for in vitro fertilization of ova from any mammalian species include development of techniques for recovery of ova that are either already competent or can attain competency for fertilization, continued development during a culture interval in vitro, and the development of means by which sperm can be adequately conditioned for fertilization. Media used for culture of ova and spermatozoa and for development of the recently penetrated ovum must be composed of the necessary factors for normal development. From experiments with rabbits, there is some evidence that a simple defined medium which supports in vitro fertilization and cleavage of ova is deficient in something that is required for continued development following embryo transfer.[16] This is not surprising, since oviductal fluid, which provides the normal milieu for preimplantation stages of pregnancy, has been shown by several investigators to change in composition as the beginnings of life progress under its influence.[17] Judicious employment of gonadotrophic hormones can be looked to as important instruments in making female gametes available. In the rabbit, recently ovulated ova can be recovered from the ovarian surface or from the oviduct. In addition, ova can be recovered from ovarian follicles just before ovulation occurs. Best in vitro fertilization results (ova fertilized/ova inseminated) are obtained by use of the most recently ovulated ova recovered from the ovarian surface,[18, 19] followed by those recovered from the oviducts,[12, 20] followed by those recovered from ovarian follicles.[14, 16] Using capacitated rabbit spermatozoa, recovered from the uterus of a mated doe, one can now expect with reasonable certainty to obtain in vitro fertilization of 80-100% of the most recently ovulated ova, 60-70% of those from oviducts, 40-50% of those from preovulatory ovarian follicles.

Sperm cells must undergo a change termed capacitation,[21, 22] which normally occurs in the female reproductive tract and which results in penetration of an ovum by the sperm cell. Sperm capacitation appears to be exaggerated in the rabbit. It seems likely that some conditioning of the sperm cells by the female reproductive tract is beneficial for successful fertilization in other mammalian species as well. It is desirable to understand the mechanism of sperm capacitation in order to duplicate this process in vitro. Capacitation of sperm can occur spontaneously in vitro in defined media in the mouse.[23, 24]   Capacitation of rabbit sperm can occur in fluids from the female reproductive tract when the proper environmental conditions are provided.[26] At least two features involved in the mechanism of sperm capacitation are recognized. These include the removal of seminal plasma components from the surface of the sperm (rabbit sperm,[26] mouse sperm,[24] ) and an increased metabolic rate as reflected by a fourfold increase in sperm respiration (rabbit sperm [27, 28] ) and motility (hamster sperm [29] ). Morphological changes in sperm cells that have become capacitated include breakdown and vesiculation of the plasma membrane with the outer acrosomal membrane, the acrosome reaction.[30]   The latter change takes place as the sperm cell passes through the surrounding cellular investments of the ovum and is now most frequently considered to follow sperm capacitation and precede sperm penetration through the zona pellucida of the ovum.

At the present time, it is possible to effect capacitation under defined in vitro conditions for epididymal sperm of the hamster[5] and the mouse.[23, 24] Sperm of different species seem to require various degrees of conditioning as reflected by the varying time intervals which they must reside in the respective female reproductive tracts before penetrating ova. Apart from this, it seems likely that the basic mechanism of sperm capacitation is similar in all mammals. Further exploitation of this hypothesis hopefully will enable the development of defined conditions for sperm capacitation useful in preparing sperm cells of many species for penetration of ova.*

---

*It may also lead to simple methods of inhibiting capacitation, hence preventing conception—Eds.

## CONCLUSION

With the realization of advances expected from continued basic research in early reproductive events, clinical application of procedures for in vitro fertilization can be predicted in human and veterinary medicine. However, a continuation of basic research in the important area of mammalian fertilization should receive even greater impetus with the approaching development of directly applicable procedures. Rapid technical improvements are anticipated in studies of extracorporeal fertilization and these advances should increase our knowledge and ability to apply such knowledge for the betterment of life for mankind.*

*The author gratefully acknowledges the support of Career Development Award HD 15861, NIH Grant RR 00340, NIH-HDO 6274-02 and a Grant from the Ford Foundation.

# References

1.  BRACKETT, B.G. Extracorporeal fertilization of mammalian ova. In *Gynecologic Endocrinology*, J.J. Gold (ed.)., Harper & Row, New York, In press.

2.  HAMNER, C.E., JENNINGS, L.L. and SOJKA, N.J. Cat (*Felis Catus* L.) spermatozoa require capacitation. *J. Reprod. Fert. 23*:477, 1970.

3.  NOSKE, I.G. In vitro fertilization of the mongolian gerbil egg. *Experientia 28*:1348, 1972.

4.  YANAGIMACHI, R. Fertilization of guinea pig eggs in vitro. *Anat. Rec. 174*:9, 1972.

5.  YANAGIMACHI, R. and CHANG, M.C. Fertilization of hamster eggs in vitro. *Nature 200*:281, 1963.

6.  EDWARDS, R.G., STEPTOE, P.C., and PURDY, J.M. Fertilization and cleavage in vitro of preovulatory human oocytes. *Nature 227*:1307, 1970.

7.  WHITTINGHAM, D.G. Fertilization of mouse eggs in vitro. *Nature 220*:592, 1968.

8.  THIBAULT, C., DAUZIER, L., and WINTENBERGER, S. Etude cytologique de la fecondation in vitro de l'oeuf de la lapine. *C.R. Soc. Biol. (Paris) 148*:789, 1954.

9.  MIYAMOTO, H. and CHANG, M.C. In vitro fertilization of rat eggs. *Nature 241*:50, 1973.

10. GOULD, K.G., CLINE, E.M., and WILLIAMS, W.L. Observations on the induction of ovulation and fertilization in vitro in the squirrel monkey (*Saimiri sciureus*) *Fert. Steril.* 24:260, 1973.

11. CHANG, M.C. Fertilization of rabbit ova in vitro. *Nature 184*:366, 1959.

12. BRACKETT, B.G. In vitro fertilization of rabbit ova: time sequence of events. *Fertil. Steril. 21*:169, 1970.

13. YANG, W.H., LIN, L.L., WANG, J.R., and CHANG, M.C. Sperm penetration through the zona pellucida and perivitelline space in the hamster. *J. Exp. Zool. 179*:191, 1972.

14. BRACKETT, B.G., MILLS, J.A., and JEITLES, G.G., Jr. In vitro fertilization of rabbit ova recovered from ovarian follicles. *Fertil. Steril. 23*:898, 1972.

15. MUKHERJEE, A.B. Normal progeny from fertilization in vitro of mouse oocytes matured in culture and spermatozoa capacitated in vitro. *Nature 237*:397, 1972.

16. MILLS, J.A., JEITLES, G.G., Jr., and BRACKETT, B.G. Embryo transfer following in vitro and in vivo fertilization of rabbit ova. *Fertil. Steril.*, 24:602, 1973.

17. BRACKETT, B.G. and MASTROIANNI, L., Jr. Composition of oviductal fluid. In *The Oviduct and Its Functions*. Johnson, D. and Foley, W. (Eds.) Academic Press, New York, In press.

18. BRACKETT, B.G., and SERVER, J.B. Capacitation of rabbit spermatozoa in a defined medium. *Fertil. Steril. 19*:144, 1968.

19.  SEITZ, H.M., Jr., BRACKETT, B.G., and MASTROIANNI, L., Jr. In vitro fertilization of ovulated rabbit ova recovered from the ovary. *Biol. Reprod. 2*:262, 1970.

20.  BRACKETT, B.G. and WILLIAMS, W.L. Fertilization of rabbit ova in a defined medium. *Fertil. Steril. 19*:144, 1968.

21.  AUSTIN, C.R. Observations on the penetration of the sperm into the mammalian egg. *Austr. J. Sci. Res. B4*:581, 1951.

22.  CHANG, M.C. Fertilizing capacity of spermatozoa deposited into Fallopian tubes. *Nature* London *168*:697, 1951.

23.  TOYODA, T., YOKOYAMA, M., and HOSI, T. Studies on the fertilization of mouse eggs in vitro. I. In vitro fertilization of eggs by fresh epididymal sperm. *Jap. J. Anim. Reprod. 16*:147, 1971a.

24.  OLIPHANT, G. and BRACKETT, B.G. Increased rate of mouse sperm capacitation utilizing media of elevated ionic strength. Presented at the Society for the Study of Reproduction meeting, Athens, Georgia, 1973.

25.  BRACKETT, G.B., MILLS, J.A., OLIPHANT, G., SEITZ, H.M., Jr., JEITLES, G.G., Jr., and MASTROIANNI, L., Jr. Preliminary efforts to capacitate rabbit sperm in vitro. *Int. J. Fertil. 17*:86, 1972.

26.  OLIPHANT, G. and BRACKETT, B.G. Immunological assessment of surface changes of rabbit sperm undergoing capacitation. *Biol. Reprod.* 9:404, 1973.

27.  HAMNER, C.E., and WILLIAMS, W.L. Effect of the female reproductive tract on sperm metabolism in the rabbit and fowl. *J. Reprod. Fertil. 5*:143, 1963.

28.  BRACKETT, B.G. Respiration of spermatozoa after in utero incubation in estrus and pseudopregnant rabbits. *VI. Cong. Intern. Reprod. Anim. Insem. Artif. Paris,* 1:43, 1968.

29.  YANAGIMACHI, R. The movement of golden hamster spermatozoa before and after capacitation. *J. Reprod. Fert. 23*:193, 1970.

30.  BARROS, C., BEDFORD, J.M., FRANKLIN, L.E., and AUSTIN, C.R. Membrane vesiculation as a feature of the mammalian acrosome reaction. *J. Cell. Biol. 34*:Cl, 1967

# PROGRESS IN MEDICAL GENETICS:
## LEGAL PROBLEMS

**Irving Ladimer, S.J.D.**

*Adjunct Associate Professor, Mount Sinai School of Medicine, City University of New York; Special Counsel/Health Care, American Arbitration Association, New York*

## THREE PERSPECTIVES ON HUMAN GENETICS

There has been an explosive increase in scientific knowledge of human genetics. The media have alerted people to the seriousness of genetic diseases and to the amazing possibilities of so-called genetic manipulation. *Legally* and *ethically*, however, there have been endless inconclusive discussions. On such basic issues as personal versus societal interests and policies regarding the population explosion in the face of limited economic resources two salient points are clear.

First, man will soon have the technical power not only to inhibit life but to modify it, and perhaps even to introduce new genetic material. Second, with the many constraints imposed by social living we will have difficulty in exercising genetic choices in ways which satisfy all.

In arriving at methods of choice, the traditional authority of the physician or scientist — the elitist, if you will — will be substantially diminished. This has developed, not only from greater dissemination and democratization of knowledge and power, but from recognition that purely technical skills are insufficient for solving human social problems.

## ISSUES AND CHOICES

In considering ethical implications, Dr. C. A. Clarke, of the Nuffield Unit of Medical Genetics, University of Liverpool, cited the following possibilities and problems suggested by modern developments in genetics.[1]

1. *Ability to detect certain abnormal fetuses early in pregnancy.* It would be ethical, Clarke maintains, to abort both probably abnormal and possibly defective fetuses, such as the male fetuses of women carrying one gene for a serious X-linked disease, such as hemophilia or the Duchenne type of muscular dystrophy.

2. *Ability to culture human cells apart from the donor.* Cells can be fused from different parts of the body or from different species. In Clarke's

view this is a valuable research method as in cancer studies. Fertilized eggs may be implanted into other tissues. Clarke considers such experiments "perfectly proper" in animals, but unethical with the fertilized human egg "until more is known about the results." In lower animals exact copies have been achieved by nuclear implants. This raises the very remote possibility that technical improvements may permit mammalian and human "cloning" or mechanical reproduction. Ramsey states "these would be an ethical problem if 'clonal man' were easy to produce" and points out the possibility of "immoral" use. [2]

3. *Ability to synthesize life in the laboratory.* Since a complete and biologically active viral chromosome can be synthesized in vitro, an extension of this work may be the manufacture of an individual human gene. Clarke comments, "I think the experiment itself is so elegant as to be equivalent to being ethical." Is this knowledge for knowledge's sake, or for its utility in replacing faulty DNA and avoiding inherited disease? The former would be a dubious ethical position. [3]

4. *Ethical problems of informing patients.* As an example Clarke mentions an autosomal dominant skin disorder, tylosis, which is itself harmless, but which is associated with the later development of cancer. He questions here whether to alert tylotic individuals to the risk of cancer and possibly to create cancer-phobia or just proceed, providing no warning to the patient of the impending danger. The underlying issue, related to telling or explaining the truth regarding any medical risk, raises legal problems of informed consent and duty to forewarn.

In general, Clarke concludes, "Advances in general come gradually and are usually unpredictable. Therefore, speculation and too detailed planning should be avoided — and bridges crossed only when they are encountered."

## THE RESPONSIBILITY OF MEDICINE

The position that detailed planning should be avoided since the future will take care of itself collides with the strong commitment for a safe, peaceful and better tomorrow.

The late George James said that medicine's principal responsibility is compassionate concern for future generations. [4] He argued for viewing and solving problems in that perspective. But what are the interests of future generations? What is a disease or a defect? How can one balance the wide range of normal and abnormal, the recognized differences in severity, possible consequences, potential for amelioration and rehabilitation, and the widespread human belief in scientific achievement? Because of such uncertainties, coercive measures should not be used even in mass screening. The welfare and freedom of individuals should come first. Thus, Dr. Robert Murray and Dr. Michael Kaback, among others, agree that it is probably unethical to mount a screening program, as for sickle cell disease, unless there are some therapeutic alternatives for patients and carriers.[5]

Paul Ramsey reminds us in discussing prenatal diagnosis, "Do no harm." Further, he says, this principle might apply to the fetus as well as to the mother.[6] Central to such right-to-life arguments are beliefs that human beings are equal and that the fetus is a person.[7] With genetic technology such as amniocentesis and elective abortion we can condemn defective fetuses, whether by counseling, social coercion, or legal requirements. Should we?

Is there some way of developing a standard for decision-making? Assuming there is a "natural" standard, which can be recognized or devised, or alternatively, that a standard set by society is to be employed, who shall apply it? The individuals involved? Does that include the newborn, the unborn, as a party? If so, how shall their interests be represented and protected? If that is to be done by society, shall it be done by social norms, law or both?

## LEGAL ISSUES

While legal and ethical concerns are intertwined, certain legal issues are clearly separable.[8] Dr. James Sorenson has suggested several legal concerns in the application of genetic knowledge.[9]

1. *Abortion*

Dr. Sorenson points out that progress in amniocentesis, in vitro fertilization, and the like are useless if they are not implemented. On January 22, 1973, the U. S. Supreme Court rendered a sweeping abortion decision in Roe V. Wade by ruling unconstitutional state laws prohibiting or restricting abortions during the first trimester of pregnancy and setting conditions for regulating or proscribing abortion procedures thereafter.[10] This decision will require modification of virtually all state abortion laws. During the first half of 1973, 13 states amended their laws to conform to prescribing conditions for performing abortions, protecting those who do not wish to take part and specifying facilities, records and other requirements.

In brief, the Court recognized three interests: privacy of the pregnant woman in the first period of pregnancy without regard to others; protection of maternal health by the State, subject to regulation; and the potentiality of human life, subject to regulation and denial of abortion, except to preserve life or health of the mother. The Court also declared the State may define "physician" and limit performance of abortions to such persons.

> Justice Blackmun wrote: "A state criminal abortion statute of the current Texas type, that excepts from criminality only a *life saving* procedure on behalf of the mother, without regard to pregnancy stage and without recognition of the other interests involved, is violative of the due process clause of the Fourteenth Amendment."

The opinion distinguishes between the protected private interests of the putative mother and those of the State:

> (a) for the first trimester, the "abortion decision and its effectuation must be left to the medical judgment of the pregnant woman's attending physician";

> (b) for the stage subsequent to the first trimester, the State, in promoting its interest in the health of the mother, may, if it chooses, regulate the abortion procedure in ways that are reasonably related to maternal health;

> (c) for the stage subsequent to viability, the State may, if it chooses, regulate and even proscribe, abortion except where it is medically determined as necessary for the preservation of the life or health of the mother.

The Court held that the general requirement that the physician use "his best clinical judgment" in arriving at an abortion decision was not unconstitutionally vague since he may decide in light of *all* attendant circumstances. Thus there are virtually no legal barriers to proposing and effecting abortion when genetic — or other reasons — may call for this option. However, *Roe* does not provide any clue as to when, in legal calculus, life begins. Thus, critics have suggested amending the Constitution to reverse or limit the opinion by some declaration of the start of life and the interest of the State in the protection of life. Dr. Alan Stone feels that the Court may have gone too far[11] since a physician may still operate to preserve the *life* or *health* of the woman at any time. Thus, the brake to be applied, if any, will respond to religious, social, or professional pressure relying on the good judgment of physicians. Historically, this represents a counter-trend; legal controls generally follow when self-determinations prove to be insufficient protection.

Although legal barriers to early abortions are now down, there still exists legal responsibility for consequences of failure to provide advice permitting a considered decision. For instance, in a genetic situation, would the physician or the hospital be legally responsible if a defective child is born? In a recent case involving a physician who erroneously advised a woman that German measles contracted during the first month of pregnancy would have no effect on her child, although he knew there was about a 25% risk, the New Jersey Supreme Court held that the defective child had no cognizable claim, because there is no remedy. To assess damages, it would be necessary, to "measure the difference between life with defects against the utter void of non-existence".[12] Such evaluation is not possible, the court said. A parallel New York case held that there is no legal remedy for having been born under a handicap "when the alternative to being born in a handicapped condition is not to have been born at all."[13] There have also been suits by a child for having been born legally a bastard because of a state hospital's failure to prevent a rape;[14] because of the father's fraudulent promise to marry the mother[15] and in other instances where there has been a charge of wrongful life.[16] Thus far, there have been no cases giving children legal rights of proper and healthy birth or non-birth. But, with opinions allowing damages to the parents for unwanted births due to defective sterilizations, the next step — recovery by the unwanted child itself — may soon follow.

### 2.   Consanguineous Marriages

Dr. Sorenson notes that there is considerable variability in state laws respecting marriage between relatives[17] for reasons of religious belief, custom, or concern for genetic consequences. Not only do the laws differ but interpretations of the same law differ markedly. The effect on any genetic control, if this is intended, will thus be most uncertain. Perhaps more serious is the growing tendency to consensual mating, that is, without any official recording or lawful establishment of a relationship.

### 3.   Marriage Between Carriers of Genetic Defects

Despite increases in genetic knowledge, there are today no legal or social constraints on marriage or mating between carriers. Screening for defects (except for PKU and, in some states, now, for sickle cell disease or trait*) is not generally mandated. In the future, the legal system might be used for compulsory screening, reporting and prohibiting carrier-carrier mating. What implications exist for privacy, for the gene pool, and for divorce? The disclosure of genetic information becomes especially critical in light of conflicting policies and cross-purposes.[18]

## 4.  *Artificial Insemination*

In recent years, artificial insemination is gaining acceptance not only in cases of sterility but also to avoid genetically defective children. The rights and duties of biological fathers and legal fathers, however, have not been established with any finality in law and decision relating to artificial insemination. The social and psychological impacts are equally not well understood. Legal clarification is obviously needed.

## 5.  *Correlation Between Chromosomal Defect and Pathologic Behavior*

One of the best examples of a modern legal genetic dilemma is the association alleged between the XYY anomaly and a predisposition to aberrant behavior. This abnormality has been advanced as a defense to charges of criminal conduct. Thus far, courts have shown no disposition to admit such an argument. Even assuming doubt about this association, does prudence suggest greater leniency for those with such conditions, special rehabilitation, or any other treatment?

On a policy level, should universal screening (including amniocentesis to detect this condition *in utero*) be imposed? Would this possibility be deemed to affect the mental health of the pregnant woman? What of the need for reports and records and the possibility that this finding might stigmatize the individual?

These considerations entwine law, social policy, private morality, and fundamental philosophic concepts of individual and community needs. True, there is no knot without the primary scientific thread suggesting a relationship, but today's scientific openness and the media promote hypotheses of this type. Misunderstandings about sickle cell trait have already led to inappropriate denials of life insurance and certain employment and hazardous exposure.

---

*Under federal law providing funds for programs, screening must be voluntary. States with compulsory laws are now changing them.

In my view, the legal process should not be employed where the facts are unclear. Against the questionable benefit of required screening and admission in a legal forum of such conditions to explain behavior, there is the definite disadvantage of stigmatization.[19]

## 6.  *Misdiagnosis and Malpractice*

Malpractice is the most obvious of all medical-legal issues. In genetic areas diagnosis rather than treatment is predominant. Negligent diagnosis, just as treatment that may lead to injury, creates liability. For genetics, including counseling and care as well as screening, standards of practice and competence must be established as the yardstick against which to measure alleged misfeasance or malfeasance. This would follow the pattern for medical and other professional activity.

So far as I know, there are no recorded cases based on legal charges of damage due to inadequate or incomplete counseling which have led to the birth of a defective child.* Although episodes in which the physician's judgment or diagnosis has been questioned or where the counseling has led to deliberate abortion of a nondefective fetus exist, I have seen no court cases brought on such accounts.

## 7.  *Experimentation*

Medical genetics raises issues common to all types of innovation in clinical practice. A major legal problem in human experimentation relates to consent and to the criteria for undertaking experiments. We rely on peer review to adjudicate the latter but there is increasing interest in including laymen in review procedures.

Informed consent and prior review are essential conditions for medical research involving human beings and are based on patients' rights to know and to participate. The report of the Department of Health, Education and Welfare Secretary's Commission on Medical Malpractice urges application of ethical guidelines for all research, regardless of auspices, including compensation for injured research subjects. Consumer participation in health care decision-making is also stressed. Extraordinary precautions should be established to protect the interest of persons not legally competent to give informed consent themselves, such as children and the mentally retarded.

---

*But, note cases based on physician and hospital misdiagnosis or improper disclosure of significance of mother's condition.[12-16]

## HOW SHALL WE PROCEED?

It is evident that this discussion has raised rather than answered questions. We need to develop purposeful, positive, and acceptable methods to permit the public, professionals, and agencies that govern and control to deal jointly and adequately with rights, obligations, and expectations raised by the "new biology".

## OBTAINING AND ASSESSING VIEWS

How can we arrive at valid opinions and an evaluation of attitudes and measure one against another?

In reviewing human studies by peer review, one method used is "risk versus benefit" analysis. It is assumed that a group of responsible peers can best estimate when and how risks will be outweighed by potential benefits.

Another decision-making mode involves translating values into social and scientific priorities. Dr. James Neel, at the 1971 Fogarty Center Conference, suggested criteria for setting priorities:[20]

1. reducing the proportion of persons with genetic disease — through prenatal diagnosis, counseling, and perhaps genetic surgery.

2. improving the expression of existing genotypes — by medical, social and nutritional measures.

3. creating genetically superior individuals — by artificial insemination or remotely by cloning.

4. protecting the present gene pool under a world policy, "that will at least ensure that as little as possible of what now exists is lost and damage through exposure to mutagens is minimized."

5. a minimum of incalculable genetic and somatic risks.

At a prior Fogarty Conference on Scientific and Ethical Considerations of Early Diagnosis of Human Genetic Defects, Neel suggested that multidisciplinary professional committees might provide advisory guidance in this field.[21] I feel that to proliferate committees and processes may be self-defeating, confusing and would leave judgment in control of the experts rather than the people. Neel considers it encouraging that the study of ethical implications in this field has come so early.

## RESOURCES AVAILABLE

Consider the institutions available to us. In an ordered society, we place great reliance on the law to require, to regulate, to sanction and to a lesser degree to stimulate and motivate action. Hence, in the interest of reducing damage or disease in our gene pool, case-law and legislation could be called on to impose screening, to prevent certain matings and to encourage certain diagnostic and identification work by limiting professional liability. It is submitted, however, that legal processes should be employed only where essential to protect the common interest and to preserve personal and private concerns. Legal strictures of course must apply to practitioners in genetic medicine to insure competent performance, on the same basis as for others, perhaps through licensure or certification.

## CONCLUSION

In summary, the multiple new problems arising from new genetic knowledge also produce legal and moral dilemmas including some unusual and novel issues. Common to their solution must be fact-finding mechanisms and devices to incorporate diverse and representative opinions and the ethical views of the community. Paramount concerns are those of privacy and the varied rights of those who cannot represent themselves effectively. Legal processes, although available, are often rigid and inflexible in the name of universality and stability. In this new field, there must be time and opportunity for experimentation and experience of personal decision. The law therefore should be applied with great restraint.

## References

1.  CLARKE, C.A. Problems raised by developments in genetics. In *Biology and Ethics*, (F. J. Ebling, editor), London and New York, Academic Press, p. 63, 1969.

2.  RAMSEY, P. *Fabricated Man: The Ethics of Genetic Control*. New Haven, Conn., Yale University Press, 1970.

3.  RAMSEY, P. "Shall We 'Reproduce'?" II. Rejoinders and future forecast. *J.A.M.A., 220:* 1480-5, 1972.

4.  JAMES, G. Clinical research in achieving the right to health. New Dimensions in Legal and Ethical Concepts for Human Research, (I. Ladimer, cons. editor), *Ann. N.Y. Acad. Sci.*, 169:301, 1970.

5.  FRANKEL, M. S. *Genetic Technology: Promises and Problems*, Monograph No. 15, Program of Policy Studies in Science and Technology, George Washington University, Washington, D. C., March, 1973.

6.  RAMSEY, P. Screening: An Ethicist's View. In *Ethical Issues in Human Genetics: Genetic Counseling and the Use of Genetic Knowledge*, (B. Hilton, et al., editors), New York and London, Plenum Press, pp. 147-161, 1973.

7.  KASS, L. R. Implications of prenatal diagnosis for the human right to life. In *Ethical Issues in Human Genetics*, ibid., pp. 185-200.

8.  CAPRON, A. M. Legal rights and moral rights. In *Ethical Issues in Human Genetics*. ibid., pp. 221-244.

9.  SORENSON, J. R. Social aspects of applied human genetics. *Social Science Frontiers*, 1971, No. 3, New York, Russell Sage Foundation.

10. ROE, et al. V. WADE, 93 S. Ct. 705, 35 L. Ed 2d 147; DOE V. BOLTON, 93 S. Ct. 739, 35 L. Ed 2d 201 (1973)

11. STONE, A. A. Abortion and the supreme court: What now? *Modern Medicine* 41:32-35, 1973.

12. GLEITMAN V. COSGROVE, 49, N.J. 22, 227 A2d 689 (1967). See Kilbrandon, Lord, The comparative law of genetic counselling. In *Ethical Issues in Human Genetics. op. cit.* pp. 245-259; SADLER, BLAIR, L. The Law and the Unborn Child: A Brief Review of Emerging Problems. In HARRIS, M. (editor) *Early Diagnosis of Human Genetic Defects — Scientific and Ethical Considerations*, Fogarty International Center Proceedings No. 6, U.S. Government Printing Office, pp. 211-229, 1972; LADIMER, I. Risks in the practice of modern obstetrics: A legal point of view. In ALADJEM, S. (editor). *Risks in the Practice of Modern Obstetrics*. St. Louis, C.V. Mosby Co., pp 246-270, 1972.

13. STEWART V. LONG ISLAND COLLEGE HOSPITAL, 296 NYS 2d 41 (1968). Here, the trial court awarded $10,000 to the mother and $100,000 to the defective child. The intermediate court, relying on *Gleitman, ibid., Williams* and *Zepeda* (see below) nullified the child's award, but retained the mother's on grounds of non-disclosure. The Court of Appeals then held that the doctors and hospital were not negligent in absence of standards regarding abortion. 238 N.E. 2d 616 (1972).

14. WILLIAMS V. STATE OF NEW YORK, 18 NY2d, 481, 223 N.E. 2nd 343 (1966).

15. ZEPEDA V. ZEPEDA. 41 Illinois. App. 2d 240, 190 N.E. 2d 849 (1963).

16. TEDESCHI, G. On tort liability for "wrongful life". *Israel Law Review, 1*:529, 1966.

17. FARROW, M. G. and JUBERG, R. C. Genetics and laws prohibiting marriage in the United States, *J. A. M. A., 209*:534-538, 1969.

18. Disclosure of genetic information: An invitational symposium. *J. Reprod. Medicine:* Lying In, 2, No. 5:211-230, 1969.

19. SHAH, S. A. (editor) *Report on the XYY Chromosome Abnormality,* Report of National Institute of Mental Health, Public Health Service Pub. No. 2103, U. S. Government Printing Office, 1970; see also FRANKEL, *op. cit.,* pp. 73-76.

20. NEEL, J. Social and scientific priorities in the use of genetic knowledge. In *Ethical Issues in Human Genetics op. cit.,* pp. 353-367.

21. NEEL, J. Ethical issues resulting from prenatal diagnosis. In *Early Diagnosis of Human Genetic Defects. op. cit.,* pp. 219-229.

# PROGRESS AND PROBLEMS IN MEDICAL GENETICS: DISCUSSION

**Dr. Walbot:** I am Dr. Virginia Walbot, Department of Biochemistry, University of Georgia. Dr. Brackett, when do you think the technology for fertilizing and implanting a human embryo will be fully developed? Given the 10 percent success rate you now have in your best system, the rabbit system, how would you superovulate human females in order to obtain enough ova to do the experiments? Lastly, do you think there are sufficient medical or clinical applications of this technique to justify research on human beings?

**Dr. Brackett:** In answer to your basic question, I am unable to predict an exact date for full development of adequate technology which would enable fertilization to take place in vitro and subsequent implantation of the resulting embryo in a human clinical situation. I expect rapid technical developments in handling of mammalian gametes, including in vitro fertilization, embryo storage, and transplantation of embryos in domestic animals, especially in the cow. Among the reasons for more rapid development of these procedures for veterinary, rather than human, clinical usage, are greater economic considerations and the absence of ethical considerations that must be resolved in development of such procedures for human use.

In response to your question regarding superovulation of human females in order to obtain enough ova to carry out such experiments I can say that many physicians around the world are using gonadotropins to treat human patients, and these treatments are effective in developing large ovarian follicles. Efforts have been made by English scientists to obtain preovulatory ova from human patients for in vitro fertilization. Following insemination of oocytes obtained in this way, they have observed cleavage stages and development as advanced as the blastocyst in two instances.

In answer to your last question, I personally believe that research on human ova and spermatozoa is justified by the potential importance of information that can be anticipated from such research. Definitive findings regarding the fertilization process must be extended ultimately to the human in order to confirm observations made in laboratory species. The value of such experiments would be to learn more about fertilization in order to enhance or inhibit union of the gametes as desired for contraception or treatment of infertility. I feel that research on human gametes is justified but much more basic research involving animal species should be done before in vitro fertilization is used as a clinical treatment for infertility of human patients.

**Dr. Walbot:** So that by using relatively immature follicles, there is a possibility of *in vitro* fertilization of human beings. Does that require an operation?

**Dr. Brackett:** Yes.

**Dr. Walbot:** In a particular individual, could the technique be applied more than once?

**Dr. Brackett:** Yes, it could be applied more than once. The procedure is usually done now by laparoscopy.

**Mark Frankel:** I am Mark Frankel, George Washington University. How far are we in development of an in utero test for a homozygote or heterozygote for sickle cell hemoglobin?

**Dr. Kaback:** There are several laboratories which have corroborated the work of Drs. Hollenberg, Kazazian and myself from Johns Hopkins[1] which showed that between the 10th and 20th week of gestation as little as 10 microliters of fetal blood could suffice to ascertain the sickle genotype. Similar methods could detect other beta chain abnormalities as well.

The problem with this early work is that all these studies were done on electively aborted fetuses. None of the work was done *in utero*. This method could detect sickle cell anemia in the fetus during the second trimester of pregnancy, if we had a method for obtaining 10 microliters of fetal blood. Amniocentesis permits one to sample amniotic fluid and its component cells, but these are not adequate for hemoglobin diagnosis. Accordingly, the fetoscope or amnioscope is needed to directly visualize the fetus in utero, and under direct visualization, to safely obtain a small sample of fetal blood. I believe that soon, perhaps in a year or two, such techniques will be available. Then the diagnosis of sickle cell anemia *in utero* will be relatively straightforward.

**Dr. Allen:** My name is Garland Allen, Washington University in St. Louis. I am a member of Scientists and Engineers for Social and Political Action (SESPA); my field is the history of science, especially the history of 20th century genetics.

A lot of ethical problems arising from any technological advance pertain to how that advance will be used. Most advances have the potential for being either good or bad, depending upon the social environment into which they are introduced. For example, studies on plant hormonal systems over the past forty years have made possible a variety of agricultural and horticultural advances of obvious benefit to human beings. Those same studies, however, have also made possible the development of the U. S. herbicide program in Southeast Asia. It is impossible to predict how scientific and technological advances can and will be used out of context.

In the case of genetic counseling, the real questions are, who is going to be counseling whom? Using what criteria? Who is going to formulate those criteria? If counseling is carried out in a hospital, who is on the hospital staff, and what kind of community does the hospital serve? How much control do members of the community have in setting criteria for counseling?

If the counseling staff is largely white and middle class, and the patients are largely black, Puerto Rican or working class, counseling comes dangerously close to racism and elitism. White doctors advise black families (especially in poor communities) not to have children (for medical or genetic reasons) more often than they so advise white families in well-to-do white communities. Detectable genetic problems are real, of course, in both communities. But in a society where good medical treatment, especially long-term treatment, for genetic defects is difficult to obtain and expensive, medical advice is different for different economic groups.

I feel our job as scientists, doctors or teachers is equally as much to work to transform our society into a more just place as to find technical solutions to medical problems. Only if we do the former, can we assure that the latter will lead to real progress and benefit for all human beings.

**Dr. Ladimer:** I am certain that most of us would agree substantially with what you have said. The thrust of what I was trying to say earlier is that we have to include all these points of view and have to get as many kinds of people, circumstances, and conditions related to decision-making as possible. I don't think these are constant or stable so there is no set formula on how to accomplish broad representation in genetic decision-making. Therefore, I would invite the kinds of people to whom you refer to take an active role, to get onto hospital committees and be heard in connection with the type of counseling they consider useful. In this way they can help make the political as well as the social decisions affecting screening.

Also, I approve of what Dr. Kaback does in providing basic, factual information and then turning the analysis and results over as appropriately as possible to the various affected groups to determine how "best" they can be applied.

**Dr. Kaback:** I want to respond to Dr. Allen's question of how our society deals with "less-than-normal individuals".

In other countries where health systems are structured in a very different manner from the United States, the problems of the mentally or physically handicapped individual are handled in a very different fashion. That is, the society as a whole (albeit much smaller and more homogeneous) recognizes its responsibilities to provide optimum care, treatment, and health care facilities for such individuals. That responsibility is accepted and shared by the society as a whole so that the individual or family burden is greatly minimized. This is not the case in American society. You are absolutely correct. Therefore, it does raise very different issues in terms of how society interacts with technology.

One can envision an evolution of both societal attitudes and technology. The interface between the two is enormously dynamic. In view of this dynamic interface, maximum and varied input must be elicited if an "optimal" result is to be achieved.

## References

1.  HOLLENBERG, M.D., KABECK, M.M., KAZAZIAN, H.H., JR., Adult hemoglobin synthesis by reticulocytes from the human fetus at midtrimester. *Science* 174, 698, 1972.

# II. COUNSELING AND SCREENING: CHOOSING OUR CHILDREN'S GENES

# CHOOSING MY CHILDREN'S GENES: GENETIC COUNSELING

Y. Edward Hsia

*Associate Professor of Human Genetics and Pediatrics, Yale University School of Medicine; Director, Genetics Clinic, Yale-New Haven Hospital; Member Yale Task Force on Genetics and Reproduction*

## INTRODUCTION: *Is There a Choice?*

We all want our children to be lovable, capable, happy and successful. We expect them to look like us, but we want them to inherit only our strengths and not our weaknesses. We certainly want their lives to be healthy and full. None of us would wish for them a shortened, painful, or crippled existence. As you have heard, however, medical science knows not only that a certain number of children will not be born whole, but that certain star-crossed families have a predictable high risk of having children born with specific disorders. The only genetic way we know to influence our children's looks, intelligence and destiny, is by choice of our mates, since inherited characteristics are derived from both parents. There is no other known way to choose advantageous genes for our children. If, however, we were at risk of bearing children with genetic disorders, would we not want to know? Can we choose not to give our children harmful genes? How can the average couple find out about such risks? If they did know of such risks would it change their outlook and plans, particularly about having children? If families at risk did change their reproductive practices, what would be the consequences for their community and for society? The process of genetic counseling aims to give relevant genetic information to families at risk so that they can appreciate the nature and extent of such risks. Is genetic counseling reaching families who need it? Is genetic counseling successful in explaining complicated medical information to the average couple? Is genetic counseling influential in changing the family plans of many couples? How should genetic counseling be done, and by whom?[1]

The answers to these questions are of importance to our society, so that societal support for genetic counseling can be appropriately regulated. We believe our experience at the Genetics Clinic at Yale provides some preliminary answers to these questions.

## DEMANDS: *Who Need to Know?*

Of every hundred babies born, three may have obvious or readily detectable malformations of the body and limbs, vital organs, or brain. Some of these babies tragically will not survive. Others, perhaps more tragically, will survive handicapped, enfeebled, or brain-damaged. Of every hundred babies born, no less tragic are the two or more born apparently normal who will falter later with innate maladies which might impair their growth, dull their intellect, or curtail their life span. All these are burdens that families would far prefer to be spared. A young couple's hopeful expectations may be cruelly dashed by the birth of an imperfect baby. They may feel anger that it happened to them, guilt that it was their fault, and fear that they are doomed to bear only deformed offspring. The burden of a crippled child may deplete their fortunes, break up their marriage, shatter their self-esteem, and alter their whole lives. They may reject all thought of having more children, or rush to reproduce, seeking the consolation and reassurance that the birth of a normal infant might give. If their true risk of having another similarly afflicted child is small, their fears may have been for nought. If their true risk was great, they may be doubly devastated by the birth of another affected baby. Parents of children bearing innate maladies which do not become manifest for many years, may have many children before realizing that several of their children might bear such a malady. Other couples might be deterred from parenthood for fear that a familial disorder could be passed on to their children.

Couples in any of these situations need to know whether there is a true biological risk of recurrence of a given condition in their family. The need to know is not only for couples aware of a familial disorder, who need clarification; but also for those who are fearful of an imagined risk, who need reassurance; and those who are totally unaware of the existence of a real risk, who need full explanation. The need is greatest if the condition is treatable by appropriate timely intervention, or if medical science can offer a couple an option to choose their children's genes.

### *How Are They Answered?*

Optimistic advisers may tell anxious families not to worry, and to take any risk. Pessimistic ones may tell them to avoid any risk. Ignorant ones may blithely give inappropriate information or advice, or else evade questioning, possibly depriving a couple of the chance to find answers to their questions. Many families rely on sources familiar to them or accessible to them, so that genetic questions are addressed to clergy, to relatives, to advice columnists, to self-styled experts with dubious qualifications, as well as to physicians and geneticists. Some physicians are not as familiar with genetic risks as perhaps they should be, and so do not welcome genetic questions or feel uncomfortable discussing the answers. Those physicians who know may dictate a course of action, may prefer not to intervene, or may have difficulty explaining complex genetic information to lay persons. An unknown number of families therefore may obtain misinformation, or be denied referral for helpful information. A large number of families undoubtedly receive warm support and accurate sympathetic guidance about genetic risks from their own physicians. Those with inherited anemias or bleeding disorders may be satisfactorily helped by their hematologists; those with genetically determined neurological disorders by their neurologists; those with familial causes of heart disease by their cardiologists, and so forth. Recent published surveys [2, 3, 4] suggest, however, that many families who need to know about genetic choice are not given sufficient information by specialist physicians, or are given it in such a way that it is poorly understood or easily forgotten. The question "How are they answered?" still lacks an accurate answer, as does the equally important question "How many are asking?"

### Who Ask at Yale-New Haven Hospital?

Analysis of the Genetic service at Yale-New Haven Hospital showed that 177 individuals or families were seen in the thirteen-month period from September 1970 through September 1971 (See Table I). Our experience is not necessarily similar to that seen by any other genetic counseling service, but it does give an indication of the types of problems that are referred to a genetic counseling service. About one-third of the families (55) were found

### TABLE I

**Patients seen September 1970 - September 1971**

|  | Total | Surveyed | Responded |
|---|---|---|---|
| Single Gene Disorder | 55 | 41 | 30 |
| Chromosomal Anomalies | 47 | 29 | 25 |
| Polygenic Defects | 15 | 14 | 11 |
| Non Genetic and Unclassified | 60 | 47 | 34 |
| TOTAL | 177 | 131 | 100 |

to have a single mutant gene of large effect, either affecting one member, or segregating in a Mendelian pattern among family members. Over one-quarter of the families (47) had one or more members affected with a significant chromosomal abnormality. About one-tenth (15) were individuals with disorders known to be influenced by polygenic factors with relatively low risks of recurrence. The others included (10) individuals with conditions known not to have a genetic cause; (29) individuals with diseases that could not be identified as having a known recurrence risk; and (21) individuals shown to be normal and free of any genetic disease, including some with genetic disease affecting a close relative but sparing themselves.

The large proportion of families found to have no recognized genetic problem is not unreasonable, although it might not have been expected. Many physicians refer patients to us for diagnostic evaluation of problems that might be genetically determined. Often, even when the answer turned out to be that not enough was known to answer their questions, it may still have been valid for them to have asked.

The socio-economic and educational backgrounds of these patients were mixed. A disproportionate number, especially of the self-referred, were better educated, from what is usually identified as the middle class. Genetic diseases know no socio-economic barriers, however, and there were patients from every type of background, including members of the medical profession. Many of our patients did come from less sophisticated indigent backgrounds, but most of these came only because their physician had recognized or suspected a serious disorder.

### What Do They Ask?

Perhaps the real basic question is "What can you do for us, and how much will it cost?" Many families come asking: "What is wrong with our child? What does the future have in store? Can you treat this condition? Why will you not cure it?" The public often has unlimited faith in the medical profession. Some families ask "Why did it happen to us?" Most include the unspoken question "Did we do something wrong?" It has not been too unusual for a family to ask "Why are we here? Why did our doctor send us?" Therefore the questions are far more complex than simply "Will it happen again?" In fact, if we enquire, we find occasionally that their real problems may include difficulties with their own marriage, with obtaining optimal care and training for their affected child or even difficulties in coping with the demands of their other children.

At the time of this survey, few members of the public have yet become aware of what medical genetics can offer, and despite much publicity, relatively few of those at risk know to ask "Can medical genetics tell me if I have a risk of having a child with a genetic disorder? Are there tests for me, or for my unborn child? Is there a genetic counseling service that can help me to choose my children's genes?"

## SUPPLY: *How Do We Answer?*

*The Team Approach:* During this period, in the Genetics Clinic at Yale, a team approach to formal genetic counseling was evolved. This was supported by a medical service grant from the National Foundation-March of Dimes. Our approach of course included many elements common to all genetic counseling services, but we have tried some innovations that have proven to be valuable. (See Diagram)

*Intake:* It is axiomatic that correct genetic interpretation is dependent upon three types of information:

1. an accurate medical diagnosis

2. complete genealogical information about all known relatives and whether any of them have the same medical diagnosis

3. adequate knowledge of the relevant scientific literature.

In order to prepare for optimal genetic counseling, three interviews are planned. An experienced nurse-coordinator handles all initial enquiries and prepares a complete pedigree at an intake interview. She collects relevant medical reports, and information about all affected family members, from other physicians and medical centers, and presents this data to the physician geneticist for interpretation. The physician geneticist studies all this collected data, reviews the medical literature, determines whether additional tests or information is needed, such as chromosome tests on the patient or parents, and prepares accurate complete genetic information to provide the family.

The third member of the team has an equally significant role. Genetic information may not be helpful to a family ill-prepared to receive it. If the medical nature of their problem is not known or clear to them, or if they are more concerned about non-genetic aspects of their problem, such as social or financial complications, they may not be ready to listen to a discourse about mechanisms of inheritance. Furthermore, the level of their education, their

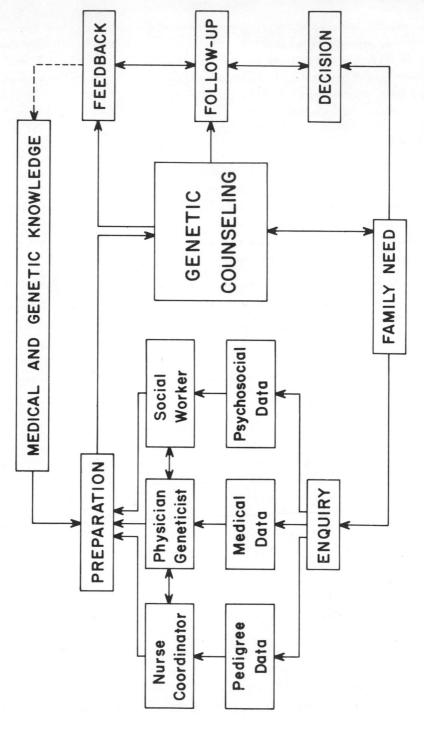

familiarity with statistical concepts of risk, and even their general vocabulary may necessitate presenting genetic information in a special way to each specific family. The third member of the team therefore is an experienced social worker, who has a third intake interview with the family to determine their true questions, whether there are other concerns, and their understanding of the medical nature of their problem. Their educational level and psycho-social background are determined, as well as their religious views, since these all influence significantly a family's attitudes toward how they might choose their children's genes.

*Output:* Adequate preparation enables the genetic counseling team to approach the counseling session with a clear plan and with confidence. Evidence of thorough preparation also gives the family more assurance that they will receive answers to their own specific questions, enabling them to approach this session with less anxiety or tension.

Accepted principles of genetic counseling are followed. We try to give a balanced understanding of the nature of the medical problem, its severity and variability, how successful treatment has been, and whether prospects for improved methods of treatment can be foreseen. We indicate the degree of confidence we have about the accuracy of the diagnosis, which family members are affected, and on what facts the diagnosis is based. We give an estimate of the recurrence risk in numerical terms, expressed both as likelihood of another child becoming affected, and likelihood of him or her being unaffected. We inform the family about availability of prenatal tests for their condition, and when applicable we describe the procedure to them. We include information about the empiric risks that all couples have of bearing a child with birth defects (3%). Our policy is to try to avoid being directive, emphasizing that the information is for their benefit, but that they have a right to utilize the information as may seem best to them, including the right to ignore it. Usually we do not tell them what other couples in their situation have done, and when asked we urge them to arrive at their own decisions. We do not ask at the counseling interview whether they have made a decision. When it seems indicated, however, we enquire whether they wish to be directed to family planning services, adoption agencies, or to special facilities for their child.

Our social worker participates in the counseling session as an objective observer and as an advocate on the behalf of the family. Her role is to ensure that the family understands what is explained, that all their special questions are considered, and to observe the effect of the counseling on the family. If necessary, she intervenes to ask discreetly for simplification or clarification, or to pose a question the family may not have vocalized. Ample opportunity is given to the family to ask questions and to discuss their concerns.

*Reinforcement:* The counseling session is concluded by reassurance that both the physician and the social worker will be available in the future to answer further questions that may arise. If other family members are at risk, they are encouraged to come for counseling too.

Finally, and probably most important, we cannot expect verbal communication to be remembered accurately, especially when unfamiliar, complicated, and emotionally laden information is presented all at once. That is why additional contact is encouraged, but the major reinforcement and follow up, in our opinion, is that we write them a letter a few weeks later summarizing the salient counseling information. If clarification of some points was necessary, or if further information needed to be presented, this was included in the written account.

The written account thus prevents misunderstanding, which is always a danger with oral communication, and reinforces their memory of the facts. It also has several other beneficial functions. It is a permanent record to which they can refer at any time, and it often contains information of vital importance to other family members to whom the letter can be shown. The family's physicians also benefit from this account, for they each receive a copy and so know exactly what was told their patients. Furthermore, the account is educational, giving genetic information to physicians and indicating how we give this genetic information to patients. In this way it is hoped that physicians will be encouraged to give genetic information to other patients with similar problems, or to refer these patients for genetic counseling too.

In the spring of 1972, we sent a questionnaire to our patients which asked whether they remembered the counseling information accurately, and whether they had made or implemented decisions about choosing their children's genes. This has also served to reinforce the genetic counseling information we gave them, allowing them again to raise more questions, and allowing us to confirm that they had indeed understood.

## QUALITY CONTROL: *Do They Understand?*

This questionnaire was sent to 131 of those who had come to us during this period (Table I, p. 45). Some mothers who had received amniocentesis during pregnancy (21), and some children suspected of having metabolic disorders such as phenylketonuria (6) were not included as they are to be part of other studies. Also, it was decided not to survey three families who had just lost a member and were in the acute grief period, and three other families who spoke no English were not included. (These families had been interviewed with interpreters, and a translation of the written account had been sent to them). Of those surveyed, one hundred replies have been analyzed.

A few respondents considered that they had already received counseling elsewhere but 90% felt that they had not. About half the respondents had had initial interviews with our social worker, of whom only seven felt it had not been of value.

They were asked what their chances were of having healthy children (Table II). Most of the answers appeared to be appropriate, but it can be seen, for example, from analysis of the 17 respondents who had had a child with Down's syndrome (Table III) that their opinions, although not necessarily wrong, differed from our judgment that the risk was not quite as good as the average couple's. Four young families were a little too optimistic.

### TABLE II

**Parental Understanding of Chances of Having a Healthy Baby**

| Response | Too Optimistic | Appropriate Answer | Too Pessimistic | Not Understood | No Answer | Total |
|---|---|---|---|---|---|---|
| Single Gene Disorders | 3 | 22 | 0 | 1 | 4 | 30 |
| Chromosomal Anomalies | 4 | 15 | 4 | 1 | 1 | 25 |
| Polygenic Defects | 1 | 8 | 2 | 0 | 0 | 11 |
| Non Genetic and unclassified | 1 | 28 | 3 | 1 | 1 | 34 |
| TOTAL | 9 | 73 | 9 | 3 | 6 | 100 |

### TABLE III

**17 Parents of Children with Downs Syndrome**

**What were their chances of having a healthy baby?**

| | Good as anyone's | Not known | Not quite as good | Definitely poorer | Not understood |
|---|---|---|---|---|---|
| Young mothers | 4 | 0 | 7 | 1 | 1 |
| Older mothers | 0 | 0 | 1 | 2 | 0 |
| Carrier mothers | 0 | 0 | 0 | 2 | 0 |

Another young family and two older families were too pessimistic. The two mothers known to be translocation carriers correctly stated their risks were significantly poorer than the average couple's. Altogether, (Table II) three-fourths of the responses appeared appropriate to us, one-tenth were too optimistic in our opinion and one-tenth too pessimistic. Three had not understood what their chances were of having a healthy child. Although asked to write down what the percentage risk of recurrence was, only a third did so, and the numerical response was inaccurate in six instances. Therefore, although the majority appeared to understand the approximate likelihood of recurrence, most families were reluctant to write down a number. Perhaps precise numerical risk meant less to them than to the counselors.

The inappropriateness of some of the responses would seem to be influenced by the severity or "burden" of the condition.[4] For instance, of the mothers of children with Down's syndrome who felt their chances of having a healthy baby were definitely poorer, one had a grown up family, the baby was not planned, and was found to have congenital heart disease. On the other hand, four of these mothers who had had a child with Down's syndrome felt their chances of having a healthy baby were as good as anyone's. This may have been because they felt that a 1% risk of recurrence was negligible; because they intended to avail themselves of prenatal diagnosis to exclude even this small risk; because we had been overly reassuring in explaining this risk to them; or because they had totally misunderstood either the counseling or the questionnaire. The burden of handicap or disease on a family is extremely difficult to weigh. Unmeasured factors such as a couple's general outlook on life, the stability of their marriage, their ultimate expectations and hopes for their children, may modify their response considerably. A mother of a child born blind was so distressed by the experience that she emphatically stated she would be unwilling to accept even a 1% risk of bearing another child with any handicap. A mother who had had several babies die at birth with gross malformations still wanted more children because the experience of pregnancy was pleasurable to her, and the loss of the affected babies was so sudden that the grief suffered was not intolerable to her. A father with one son crippled by muscular dystrophy denied the medical evidence that his younger son was going to develop the disease and refused to admit that there was any risk of recurrence for future children. We found that the severity of the condition produced highly in-dividualistic responses, some positive and some negative. The concept that the severity of a genetic disorder is a major determinant of the response of a family is certainly valid[4] but needs much careful evaluation.

Families were asked whether they felt the doctor answered all their questions satisfactorily (Table IV): 83 replied yes, 5 replied no. They were asked whether the doctors talked on a level they could understand, way over their head, or down to them. Of 95 who answered this question, only one felt the level was too high, and one felt the level was too low. When asked whether they understood what had been told to them, most felt they did understand, but three did not. Most families felt they had received a reasonable explanation to their questions. This response undoubtedly was biased by the way we asked and by the fact that it was asked by us. If we had enquired whether they understood the principles of genetics, or what a chromosome was, or if we had judged the appropriateness of their response by the accuracy of a numerical answer, they would have scored far less favorably. Our objective though was to assess whether they had retained a satisfactory grasp of the genetic risk of recurrence of the condition affecting their family, and to determine whether refresher interviews were necessary.

The appropriateness of the majority of the replies might be attributed at least in part to the value of the written account most families received. When asked what they had done with the written account (Table V), of 73

## TABLE IV

### Satisfaction, Comprehensibility and Comprehension

| Satisfactory Answers to All Questions | | More Discussion Desired | | Level of Discussion | | Did They Understand? | |
|---|---|---|---|---|---|---|---|
| Yes | 83 | Satisfied | 73 | Right | 93 | Yes | 76 |
| No | 5 | More desired | 9 | Wrong | 2 | Partly | 5 |
| | | | | | | No | 3 |

## TABLE V

### Written Account of Genetic Counseling

| | Reread many times | Shown to relatives | Kept in safe place | Total |
|---|---|---|---|---|
| Mendelian Disorders | 8 | 8 | 14 | 20 |
| Chromosomal Anomalies | 6 | 6 | 18 | 19 |
| Polygenic Defects | 2 | 3 | 8 | 8 |
| Other conditions | 4 | 8 | 20 | 26 |
| TOTAL | 20 | 25 | 60 | 73 |

families who had received an account only one family had discarded it. A year later, this couple remembered that their child's problem had been traced to intrauterine infection with toxoplasmosis and so had no need to keep the letter (they also had decided not to have any more children and felt the service had not been worth the cost). The majority had put it away with important papers, many had read it repeatedly "to make more sense" and others had shown it to close friends and relatives.

Perhaps most significant is that only four noted that it had differed from what they remembered they had been told. The significance was because on occasion this account in fact had intentionally been written to differ in emphasis or in detail. It was used to expand some aspects of the counseling, but particularly to reemphasize the balance of the basic facts which may have become distorted at the personal interview. Despite the fact that the written account was therefore a restatement of the relevant facts, and was not necessarily a repeat of what was said at the interview, few families noted the difference. We interpret this as an indication that people's memory of an oral interview is imperfect. One respondent wrote in the margin: "I understood some of what the doctor said, but it came as such a shock that I was too upset to hear much of what he said." The more balanced effect of the written account is demonstrated by responses to the question: Did they feel the doctor had advised them to have more children (Table VI). Our intention had been to be non-directive, leaving the choice of whether to have more children up to the family. Less than one in six of those receiving a written account felt the doctors had given them directive advice. But more than one in three of those *not* receiving a written account considered that directive advice had been given.

What decisions did families make about having more children? Many had non-genetic reasons for not having more children, such as size of family,

## TABLE VI

### Family's Impression about Genetic Counselor's Advice

| Written Account | To have more children | Not to have more children | Choice up to themselves | Total |
|---|---|---|---|---|
| Sent | 6 | 4 | 52 | 62 |
| Not sent | 4 | 3 | 12 | 19 |
| TOTAL | 10 | 7 | 64 | 81 |

financial, or marital problems. Fifty-nine families did make a decision about future children based upon genetic information. Among those with chromosomal disorders (Table VII), 14 decided to have more children. Four mothers elected to have amniocentesis when they became pregnant, one mother chose not to have the procedure. The five infants born were all normal. When considered according to the size of their recurrence risk (Table VIII), 19 families, mainly with single gene disorders, had a recurrence risk of greater than 10%, and 40 families had a recurrence risk of less than 10%. A majority of those with a high risk had decided to postpone having children, and almost half of those with a low risk had decided to have more children.

Dr. C.O. Carter and his colleagues from London[5] had found 3 to 10 years after counseling that about two-thirds of 279 families with a high risk of recurrence had been deterred from having more children, and one-quarter of 311 families with a low risk of recurrence had been deterred. Our recent findings in a much smaller sample, after a shorter interval, is not very different, except that many of our families had not yet made a final decision.

### TABLE VII

#### Decisions Made about Having More Children

| Chromosomal Disorders | Decisions | | |
|---|---|---|---|
| Down's syndrome | To have more | Not to have more | To postpone decision |
| Young mothers | 10 | 2 | — |
| Older mothers | 2 | 1 | — |
| Carrier mothers | 1 | — | 1 |
| Other Chromosomal disorders | 1 | 1 | 2 |

### TABLE VIII

#### Decisions Made about Future Offspring

| | To have more children | Not to have more children | To postpone decision |
|---|---|---|---|
| High risk of recurrence ( >10%) | 4 | 5 | 10 |
| Low risk of recurrence ( <10%) | 18 | 10 | 12 |

Many other considerations affect the reproductive decisions that a family may make. Pressure or support from relatives, their own psychosocial bias, guidance or influence from their clergy or from other physicians will all modify their attitudes toward a genetic risk that has been told to them.

Decisions may be modified by the course of events and experience. For instance, we have found in our clinic that parents of a child having dietary restriction for phenylketonuria often postpone having any more children for two to four years. When they saw their child was growing satisfactorily with evidence that intelligence had been preserved, six of these parents chose to accept the 25% risk of having another similarly affected child.

Five babies have been born so far, one of these had phenylketonuria, and one hyperphenylalaninemia. Other families may postpone a decision in the hope that further scientific advances may be of help to them, or because they are reluctant to commit themselves one way or the other.

One endearing boy in our study was shown to have cystinosis. The parents, who were intelligent and well-educated, understood intellectually that life-threatening renal disease would develop in a decade, although he was the picture of health when they were counseled. They decided to take the 25% predicted risk and had another child. Unfortunately, tests on their new baby showed he too was affected. Subsequently they have decided to postpone having another child. (This family also expressed negative feelings about the genetic counseling, stating that it was not worth the cost to them).

## COST ANALYSIS: *Was it Worthwhile?*

It should be obvious by now that it is entirely false to imply in 1972 that there is any way to choose genes for one's children. Rather, the real choice is whether one should have children at all if there is a predicted risk that one's child would carry a deleterious gene or genes, or whether one should choose selectively to have children proven by prenatal tests to be unaffected by genetic or chromosomal defects. What criteria can be used to determine whether genetic counseling was worthwhile?

Diagnosis followed by successful treatment of a genetic disease would seem to be worthwhile. Forewarning of a family with a major genetic risk who then refrain from having children, or reassurance of a family with negligible genetic risk who then have more children also appears worthwhile. Reproductive decisions and practices were the criteria Dr. Carter and his colleagues used to assess whether their counseling was worthwhile. Other less objective criteria might be equally valid. If a family had been given a better understanding of the nature of their problem, even if their plans for future children remain unaltered, they may consider that they have received a worthwhile service.

In our questionnaire, we asked not only whether they had been satisfied with the counseling, but also whether they had felt it was worth the cost (Table IX). It can be seen that only 10% of those who answered felt it was not worth the cost. This data is obviously biased, because some families had medical insurance, others were on welfare, many were not charged the full fees. Even allowing for these factors, over half of all the 131 surveyed, and 90% of those who answered this question, felt that the cost was worth whatever they had been asked to pay.

The cost to each individual family perhaps should be considered also in terms of what their response to this expensive service should be. Does the family receiving genetic counseling have an obligation to utilize the genetic information that has so painstakingly been given to them?

My own view is that each family has a right to health facilities, and, if there is relevant genetic information, it should be made available to them. I see no conflict between this view and the view that every one has a right to utilize this information or to ignore it. The precious birth-right of individuals in our society includes the right to choose our mates by mutual agreement and the right to procreate if physically and medically possible. Unfavorable genetic information may deter a family from exercising their right to procreate, but it is their right to choose whether to have children even if they cannot choose their children's genes.

### TABLE IX

#### Was Genetic Counseling Worth the Cost?

|                        | Yes | No |
| ---------------------- | --- | -- |
| Mendelian Disorders    | 13  | 3  |
| Chromosomal Anomalies  | 19  | 2  |
| Polygenic Defects      | 10  | 0  |
| Other conditions       | 28  | 2  |
| TOTAL                  | 70  | 7  |

## PROJECTION: *What Should You Do?*

If genetic counseling is worthwhile, and is of benefit to most of those who ask, we as individual members of society have at least a moral obligation to encourage and support genetic counseling services. If the services are too complicated and costly to become readily available to all who need it, society has a right to demand that the cost be reduced.

The cost can be reduced by improving the efficiency of genetic counseling. If our school children are given a better understanding of genetic mechanisms in biology, eventually fewer of them will need to receive individual genetic instruction the way it is presented at Yale. If, by surveys and analysis of studies like the present one, parts of the genetic counseling service is found to be of lesser value, these parts can be de-emphasized or eliminated so that the essential elements of genetic counseling can be presented more efficiently. If these essential elements can be given by physicians to meet the needs of their patients, or if non-medical geneticists can readily be trained to give these elements of genetic counseling, the service can economically be made available to many more families.

These objectives imply that some form of quality control is required, and either professional self-regulation, or some form of societal regulation of the quality of genetic counseling should be established to ensure that families receive accurate information, suitable for their needs.

Societal responsibility perhaps should also regulate the response of individual families. Perhaps the individual right to procreation must be restricted. If a family has a major risk of bearing children with major genetic deficiencies, it is not only a tragedy for the individual and the family, but society may have to shoulder a major share of the medical and social cost of caring for such an individual. If such a family should choose to ignore the risk, and continue to procreate, the cost to society will be multiplied by the birth of each affected individual. In such a situation, can society take upon itself the right to limit the number of children such a family might bear? Can society insist upon prenatal detection tests or on appropriate preventive treatment for affected individuals? These become public health measures analogous to the right of a community to restrict the movements of an individual with a highly contagious disease such as smallpox. Genetic diseases are not contagious, but they are transmissible. What should you do? [6, 7]

# References

1.  HECHT, F., HOLMES, L.B. What we don't know about genetic counseling. *New Engl. J. Med., 287*: 464-465, 1972.

2.  EMERY, A.E.H., WATT, M.S., CLARK, E.R. The effects of genetic counseling in Duchenne muscular dystrophy. *Clin. Genet., 3*: 147-150, 1972.

3.  REISS, J.A., MENASHE, V.D. Genetic counseling and congenital heart disease. *J. Pediat. 80*: 655-656, 1972.

4.  LEONARD, C.O., CHASE, G.A., CHILDS, B. Genetic counseling, a consumer's view. *New Engl. J. Med., 287*: 433-439, 1972.

5.  CARTER, C.O., FRASER ROBERTS, J.A., EVANS, K.A., BUCK, A.R. Genetic clinic: A follow-up. *Lancet, 1*: 281-285, 1971.

6.  This study has been made possible only because of the genetic counseling given by my colleagues, Drs. L.E. Rosenberg, M.J. Mahoney, T.D. Gelehrter and W.R. Breg, and because of the unstinting contributions to genetic counseling at Yale of our nurse-coordinator, Mrs. A. Waters and our social-worker, Mrs. R. Silverberg.

7.  This work was supported in part by a National Foundation Medical Service Grant #C-41 and PHS training grant HD-00198-06.

# GENETIC COUNSELING: SOME PSYCHOLOGICAL CONSIDERATIONS

### James R. Sorenson

*Associate Professor of Socio-Medical Sciences, Boston University School of Medicine, Boston, Massachusetts.*

Within recent years a few articles have appeared which examine some possible consequences of applied human genetics in the context of genetic counseling, [1, 2, 3, 4, 5, 6]  These articles have explored genetic counseling in two senses also apparent in Dr. Hsia's presentation. They are first, the level of *understanding* achieved by genetic counseling clients and the amount of information clients retained after various periods of time and second, the attitudinal and actual reproductive *behavior* of clients subsequent to counseling. Since most counselors take as their goal in genetic counseling the provision of sufficient information to enable clients to make rational decisions about future reproduction, it is understandable why they have examined these two topics.

Much more is involved in genetic counseling than the provision of scientific and medical information. Considerably more can result from genetic counseling than just changes in reproductive attitudes and behavior. To explore these effects it will prove useful to introduce another dimension into the discussion. This dimension involves essentially the personal *meaning* attached to individual experiences with genetic problems or, to phrase it differently, the psychological and social hazards associated with genetic counseling. These can be divided into three large categories.

First, genetic counseling involves for many individuals the first realization, and for most affected patients initial expert confirmation that they personally carry a genetic defect and are, therefore, somehow different from most people. In so doing, counseling may provide a basis, first of all, for personal stigmatization and the psychological problems associated with stigmatization. Second, in many cases it appears that counseling can pose a threat to the close interpersonal relations of a client. Most counseling today involves couples, and the labeling of either one or both as genetically defective may entail significant alterations in the equilibrium of a marriage. Finally, genetic counseling can bring to a couple their first realization of what the chances are that they may never have a healthy child, and thus, that they may never fulfill the societal role of normal parenthood. Such a situation can pose problems of adjustment for a couple and distinguishes them as a family unit.

## PERSONAL IDENTITY AND GENETIC COUNSELING

It appears that by far the most common situation in counseling involves a couple arriving at the counseling clinic subsequent to the birth of a defective child, seeking information prior to having a second one. Our research at Princeton indicates that 80 percent of genetic counseling clients appear under these circumstances.[7] In England, Carter provides data which indicate that 92 percent of the couples in his study fall into this category,[1] and Leonard and associates at Johns Hopkins report that the majority of couples in their study of genetic counseling had only one afflicted child.[2]

Many parents have very poor knowledge of their problem prior to counseling. In most cases this leaves them ill-prepared for the information conveyed in the counseling situation. As parents of a defective child, they already carry the burden of what can be called a courtesy stigma.[8] By this we mean that they are regarded by others generally as different because they share a web of affiliation with the stigmatized, and as such, as Birenbaum has noted in his research on parents of mental retardates, they occupy an ambiguous place in society.[9] On the one hand, such persons are still normal, that is, they are not visibly abnormal, but in another sense, a biological or parental sense, they are now different.

The psychological threat of being labeled genetically defective can pose many problems for counselees and counselors. While there is not a great amount of literature on these problems, what does exist suggests that psychological problems in accepting genetic information about oneself and one's children are not small for a significant number of people. Leonard and associates report that of the 61 couples surveyed in their study, nearly 50 percent reported one or another type of problem in receiving and understanding information conveyed in counseling.[2] Five of their families indicated that they had never been counseled, even though they had. In another six families the parents expressed denial by not accepting certain aspects of the counseling. Five more families reported that they were in such a state of emotional shock that they could not remember what was said in counseling. Nine additional families reported inability to understand the counseling or to apply it in a meaningful way to their situation.

Reiss and associates, in a recent study of genetic counseling and congenital heart disease, found that of the 35 couples only 9, or about 21 percent, could remember the potential recurrence risk to subsequent off-spring when questioned one to four months after being told.[3] This was so even though these couples had expressed interest in such information. Hsia and his colleagues at Yale report that they have experienced a much higher level of genetic client comprehension with only 27 percent of their 100 clients reporting misinformation or no understanding.[4]

The available literature thus suggests that anywhere between 21 and 75 percent of clients who go through counseling report difficulty in remembering or acquiring genetic information. Certainly, a significant portion of this is due in part to the psychological distress and disorientation clients can experience. The provision of advice in counseling, when seen from the perspective of the counseling client, involves not only the acquisition of information, but often necessitates changes in certain aspects of the self-image, a process requiring time, psychological adjustment and perhaps considerable personal effort. As such, it is not surprising that there are communication problems in counseling and that many clients distort, forget, or reject the scientific information conveyed by the expert in genetics.

## INTERPERSONAL RELATIONS AND GENETIC COUNSELING

There are scant data to indicate the family problems which might accrue from genetic counseling. Carter and his associates report that the incidence of divorce among all their genetic counseling couples three to ten years after counseling was no higher than the rates for comparable age cohorts in England at that time.[1] Two comments may place this observation in perspective.

First, divorce, while becoming socially more acceptable, is still frowned upon in Western culture, and there is considerable social pressure for couples to maintain a legal marital unit even if facing severe problems. Perhaps more importantly, divorce reflects the most extreme social announcement of problems, and the lack of divorce implies little, if anything, about the satisfaction that couples (may in fact) experience in a marriage.

Second, a close examination of Carter's data reveals that, although for his couples in general the rate of divorce was normal, the rate among those who reported that counseling had changed their reproductive expectations was three times the national average.[1] For those couples for whom counseling meant something, for whom it altered reproductive careers, a much higher proportion obtained divorces or were separated than is statistically normal. For couples who reported no effect of counseling on their reproductive expectations, there were normal or below normal levels of divorce. While these data are limited, they suggest that counseling may lead not only to changes in reproductive plans but also to changes in reproductive partners.

The disclosure of genetic responsibility can pose many problems for couples, and genetic counselors are aware of this. For example, genetic counselors sometimes present information in the counseling situation in such a way that they do not tell the couple everything. Rather, they construct the scientific information so that a couple, in all likelihood, will not deduce the fact that one is in fact genetically responsible for the disease that their child has or for the risk that they face should they tempt fate again. Stevenson and colleagues in noting the problems inherent in designating genetic responsibility in one parent write,

> It seems wise, unless it is obvious to patients or necessary for some reason, not to indicate that a condition was inherited through one or the other parent, as this can be a source of marital friction.[10]

By diffusing responsibility, not by constructing a fabrication but by carefully presenting their information, counselors, in the traditional role of the doctor, are revealing their concern with the total patient. At the same time, they are recognizing that disclosure of genetic status might have significant effects on an established marriage.

## THE NUCLEAR FAMILY AND GENETIC COUNSELING

The data on parental reproductive behavior subsequent to counseling are perhaps the most interesting. While the data are limited and somewhat inconsistent, they provide some opportunity to explore the many problems and issues that parents facing a potential genetic problem must consider.

The largest body of data on reproductive behavior is reported by Carter and his colleagues in England.[1] They followed 421 couples three to ten years after they had received counseling. Defining a high recurrence risk as one of 1 in 10 or greater, they found that about two-thirds of the couples in this situation were deterred as a result of genetic counseling, whereas about one-fourth of the couples facing a risk of less than 1 in 10 was deterred. It should be noted that these figures refer to what couples said was the impact of genetic counseling on their intentions not to their actual reproductive behavior. These data suggest that counseling can have a very significant impact on reproductive attitudes. The data also suggest that the degree of risk which a couple faces is a significant and potent factor shaping these self-reported attitudes.

Hsia, in his Yale study, also reports on client reproductive attitudes subsequent to counseling. His data indicate that approximately 25 percent of the couples with a high risk were deterred by counseling, and that nearly an equal proportion were deterred among the low-risk group.[4] This is much lower than the percentage noted by Carter.

If we turn our attention now to the actual reproductive behavior of couples as reported by the Carter data, the following patterns emerge. First, of those parents facing a high risk and stating that they were attitudinally deterred by genetic counsel, 24 percent had at least one additional pregnancy. Of those facing a smaller risk, but also stating that they were attitudinally deterred, 15 percent had at least one additional pregnancy. The comparable crude reproductive figures for couples not deterred attitudinally by genetic counseling were 85 percent and 87 percent respectively. If the Carter data are combined so that we look only at actual reproductive behavior subsequent to counseling as a function of whether a couple faced a high or low risk the following picture emerges. Of those couples confronting a one in ten risk or greater, fully 46 percent had at least one additional child, while for those facing a smaller risk, 70 percent had one additional child. These data suggest that there is considerable variance between the effects of genetic counseling in terms of its impact on the attitudes and actual reproductive behavior of couples.[1] Counseling seems to affect attitudes more than actual reproductive behavior.

## CONCLUSION

In reviewing the available data, it becomes apparent that a number of problems of communication exist. Couples may fail to understand what the counselor explains, they may not translate the information into expected attitudes, or their behavior may be inconsistent with their professed attitudes. Counseling may be traumatic and emotional trauma may interfere with the patients comprehension or ability to act on what is comprehended. A significant proportion of counseled couples have an additional child even when they have altered their contraceptive behavior. Thus, for such recipients of counseling, more is involved then hearing the estimated recurrence risks.

The point of this discussion is not to negate the importance of the impact of recurrence risk and the sense of disease burden on reproductive attitudes and behavior. Rather, it is to point out that reproductive behavior takes place in a social context. The information presented to a couple in genetic counseling is not the only factor determining their attitudes and behavior. With adoption lessening as an available option to couples* facing genetic disaster, and with many, if not most, finding artificial insemination at variance with their personal and cultural conceptions as to the social and biological integrity of the family, many find themselves in an extremely anxiety-provoking situation. The available data have been collected almost totally on couples who already have one afflicted child. In these couples, perhaps even more so than in those who know one and/or the other spouse carries a bad gene and who have not yet had any children, the desire for a normal child can be very great. Whatever the case, the fact remains that a significant proportion of couples facing genetic problems with a high recurrence risk and with marked personal burden, consciously or unconsciously, gamble on having a normal child. To more fully evaluate the impact of genetic counseling as it is now practiced, it is necessary that future studies orient themselves to the effects of counseling on families with and without healthy children, on families with ethnic traditions stressing large families, and on other social and psychological factors which may significantly affect the manner in which genetic counseling clients interpret, accept, and act on the information and advice they receive in the genetic counseling session.

---

*At the same time adoption has become more difficult as a result of the reduction in unwanted births, it has also become more acceptable as concern for population control has become widespread—Eds.

# References

1.  CARTER, C., EVANS, K., FRASER-ROBERTS, J.A. and BUCK, A. Genetic clinic: A follow-up, *Lancet, 1*:281-285, 1971.

2.  LEONARD, C., CHASE, G., and CHILDS, B., Genetic counseling: A consumer's view, *New Engl. J. Med. 287*:433-439, 1972.

3.  REISS, J.A., MENASHE, V. Genetic counseling and congenital heart disease. *J. Pediat., 80*:655-656, 1972.

4.  HSIA, Y.E. Choosing my children's genes: Genetic counseling, pp. 43-59, this volume.

5.  CARTER, C., Comments on genetic counseling, *Proceedings of the Third International Congress of Human Genetics,* 97-100, 1966.

6.  SMITH, C., HOLLOWAY, S., and EMERY, A., Individuals at risk in families with genetic disease. *J. Med. Genet. 8*:453-459, 1971.

7.  SORENSON, J. *Final report: Applied human genetics planning study.* (unpublished manuscript) Princeton University, 1971.

8.  GOFFMAN, E. On cooling the markout, *Psychiatry, 15*:451-463, 1952.

9.  BIRENBAUM, A. On managing a courtesy stigma, *J. Health and Soc. Behav., 11*:196-206, 1970.

10. STEVENSON, A.C., DAVIDSON, B.C., and OAKES, M.W. *Genetic Counseling,* Philadelphia, J.B. Lippincott Co., 1970.

# DOWN'S SYNDROME IN THE FAMILY:
# A PERSONAL PERSPECTIVE

**Mrs. Hubert H. Humphrey**
*Washington, D.C.*

As the grandparent of a 12-year-old girl with Down's syndrome, I know fully the importance of counseling to parents who are heartbroken by the birth of a handicapped child and fearful of having other children. More than anything else, they need information. They need to know that there will be professional support available to help them in the days, months and years ahead and genetic counseling to determine the advisability of having other children.

We concentrate our attention so frequently on how parents and other family members respond to the birth of the handicapped child that we forget it may be more important how the professionals respond; the doctor, the nurse, the social worker — how they tell the parents, how they feel toward the child, the terminology that is used in conveying the sad news, how they interpret the future.

I remember when Vicky (our granddaughter) was born that one of the doctors stopped me in the hospital corridor and abruptly said, "What do you know about mongolism?"

My first thought was, "Does he mean our baby? What does mongolism have to do with our new baby?" My mind went racing back to my college psychology days. I recalled the words "idiocy" and "moron". The world suddenly stopped.

Later, after careful examination of Vicky, there was a conference with the doctors at the hospital. The gynecologist urged us to consider institutional care. But the pediatrician would make no recommendation on this. He frankly said that there were pros and cons to be carefully considered.

As I listened to the optimistic report on her physical health, my mind quickly projected into the future — into the many years ahead. I knew the experience of parents who had children who needed to be looked after far into adulthood and the tremendous drain it had been on them and the other members of their family. I could not put aside a feeling of deep despair.

Then I heard the pediatrician saying, "She will undoubtedly be happier than you are about the situation as a parent or grandparent. She will be happier than the normal child." I remember this being a comforting thought.

But you awake the next morning and there it is — the emptiness, the knowledge of tragedy, as though you had just lost a dear member of the family. The telephone calls were an immediate problem. What do you answer when someone says, "We are so happy you have your granddaughter. How is she?"

Here we were people who were informed on so many problems. Hubert and I had visited health facilities all over the world. Physical and mental handicaps were not new to us. And yet we felt so helpless in this situation, so needful of enlightened guidance.

How would my daughter and her husband feel about their decision regarding their child's care in a week, a month, a year from now? How would we feel about it? What would Vicky be like at two, at eight, at 16, at 40?

The doctors and other professionals we consulted tried hard to provide us with the answers we sought. But we found that most of them had encountered the mongoloid child and other types of mentally retarded persons infrequently. Most often, as in our case, this had been only in the hospital setting. The doctors, especially, often did not know what happened once the child went home with parents or to a residential facility.

While they had previously recommended institutional care for families, they had seldom, if ever, visited the facilities themselves. Medical school courses had only briefly touched on the problem.

My daughter convinced her husband to bring to the hospital her pediatrics book from her nursing school course. And in that volume she read misinformation that her own doctors had already discounted — that the mongoloid child was not likely to live past the age of 12.

Of course, I find more enlightenment today as far as the mentally retarded are concerned than when our granddaughter was born but still not enough to keep me from prodding those who bear the great responsibility for providing diagnostic help and assisting with proper planning for the handicapped child's care. So there is much yet to do. The work is far from finished.

In the area of genetic counseling, I suspect that the greatest problem, particularly in other than affluent America, is the lack of awareness of this service and the assistance it can be to parents with special problems. I know my mail reflects this. Thus, those who work in this field have a responsibility to educate and to assure that this newfound knowledge is within the reach of all who need it.

# THE RIGHT TO CHOOSE OR TO IGNORE

**Harvey Bender, Ph.D.**

*Professor of Biology, Notre Dame University*

Like politics, genetic counseling is the art of the possible rather than an ideal abstraction. It is essential then to first consider the current state of the art. The genetic counselor today is not a genetic engineer. Rather, he addresses himself to the identification of genetic disorders and those individuals capable of transmitting those disorders. He is primarily interested in prevention, and in those relatively few areas in which our knowledge is adequate, in treatment and possible cure. Despite the remarkable advances in medical and human genetics in the past few years, genetic counseling is still a new, incomplete, rapidly expanding field.

## A MODEL FOR GENETIC COUNSELING

But genetic counseling is nevertheless the most significant resource we now have for direct human intervention in choosing our children's genes. To assess the impact of genetic counseling, a model can be drawn from observations of existing programs. Despite their variability, there are certain constants. The genetic counseling process can be divided into diagnostic, educational, and decision-making components.

Today, the counselor assumes responsibility for both diagnosis and education.* The crucial stage, the process of actual choice, is left to the individual. The counselor is scrupulously careful not to impose a decision upon the client.

## VALUES IMPLICIT IN THE
## USUAL COUNSELING MODEL

Yet this model is clearly not value-free. First, it presupposes both implicitly and explicitly the desirability of making genetic choices. It also places a premium on self-awareness and self-discipline. Thus, it is designed to maximize the possibility for responsible choice by the involved individual himself. It institutionalizes one of this society's fondest values: the belief in the individual's right to know and to choose.

---

*Some groups separate these functions—Eds.

## PROBLEMS IN THE PRACTICE

First, there is failure of the clients ability to benefit. The gap between specialized knowledge and public information is so extreme that not all those who need counseling know that they need it. Many who do know, do not know how to obtain it. Those who find their way into counseling facilities are often so unsophisticated about genetic counseling, and even genetics itself, that they do not actually understand why they are there or the benefits which may accrue. This process thus shows extraordinary faith in both the institution and the referring agent, be he the family physician, minister, or concerned friend. Given such innocence it seems questionable to assume that the individual today is in a position to regulate his own genetic future.

Second, there are problems in the institutionalization of counseling especially concerning costs. The cost of concerned and thorough counseling is high. Since society must bear the cost of the genetically impaired — both immediately, in its institutions and agencies, and in the future, in terms of the alteration of the gene pool — some suggest society ought to bear the costs of counseling: an economy in this larger perspective.

But how can society be expected to arrive at such a decision? If understanding is so inadequate that even some clients who appear for counseling do not comprehend its value or implications, how can society in general cogently choose to assume the costs of genetic counseling? It is even more difficult to imagine society's imposing any sort of controls to enforce counseling decisions. Indeed, many regard attempts by society to enforce ethical choices as encroachment on the individual's rights to know and to choose — and to choose not to choose.

Further, as counselors and educators, we are profoundly concerned with the ethics and morality of controlled genetic choice — who shall decide, on what basis, for whom? But a public which does not have the basic data for the limited genetic choice possible today cannot address itself intelligently to these questions. As the possibilities become more complex, choice will be more difficult.

## THE RIGHT TO CHOOSE

The counseling model, which affirms the individual's right to choose, is also predicated upon his right to know and his ability and willingness to act. This creates an interesting dilemma in the light of our current social and moral debate.

As a society, and specifically in genetic counseling, we place our highest value on a structure which least restrains individual behavior. Yet we have been unwilling to commit our social resources to research and education in order to make individual choice meaningful.

Certainly, we can cite instances in which education of the individual leads to his making responsible choices, especially if he is offered and can afford technological and social means to implement that choice. For example, the population debate, plus birth-control technology, may have led individuals to choose to adopt a system of birth regulation. The ecologists' projections, adequate facilities, and social sanctions induce some of us to recycle newspapers and use public transportation.

But these decisions are made by a minority of individuals. It is a quantum leap to imagine mass acceptance of such values and widespread social decisions based on and reinforcing such values. Such decisions indeed would signal a new awareness of the interdependence of individual and societal rights.

## THE RIGHT NOT TO KNOW

In fact, quite another pattern, which sharply conflicts with the right-to-know-plus-ability-to-act model we have outlined, seems to be emerging today. It is the craving to assert a right NOT to know. It is part of a wave of anti-scientific, anti-technological sentiment prevalent in the early seventies.

Some problems related to the sickle cell anemia screeening programs provide a cogent example. The immediate results of the testing program, its impact felt on job possibilities and insurance rates for identified afflicted blacks, have cause a screening backlash. There is widespread ignorance and confusion about the ultimate benefits of such screening. The immediate is visible and the future seems problematic. Thus people demand the right not to know about their genetic problems — or at least would insist not to let society know, claiming an unjustifiable invasion of privacy.

John Maddox's recent book *The Doomsday Syndrome* indirectly provides support for this apparently basic desire not to know. The public today — perhaps understandably — shrinks from the enormous burden of solving the crises the futurists project. Unwilling to commit themselves psychologically or economically, some people would far rather gain a reprieve from such responsibility and settle for an uneasy truce with the *status quo*.

At best, assertions of the right not to know may buy time. But the real costs of the delay, individual and social, are incalculable. By putting off difficult decisions today, we may force far more drastic decisions in the future. By asserting our individual freedom, we may jeopardize it.

The right not to know is likely to become an evermore important factor in the area of genetic testing and counseling and must be considered in relationship to our counseling model.

A society which chooses not to know, through reluctance to assume the costs of counseling, basic research, and effective public education, has made — whether it knows it or not — a significant ethical and moral decision. Society's current desire not to know is in mortal combat with one of its most cherished values: the right of the individual to make responsible choices and take appropriate action.

# COUNSELING AND SCREENING: DISCUSSION

**Dr. Jemison:** I am Evelyn W. Jemison, Director of the Sickle Cell Program and Associate Professor of Biology, Virginia State College, Petersburg, Virginia. I am very much concerned about the psychological impact of sickle cell information on non-blacks that has produced increased stigmatization of the black school children in Virginia. Why is it that the heterogeneity of the United States population does not result in the testing of all sub-populations, as in the case of PKU testing? Is this in any way a prejudicial bias? Are there any published data that relate to the psychological impact of testing and screening programs on both blacks and non-blacks?

**Professor Sorenson:** Unfortunately, my answer may reflect only my lack of knowledge of relevant literature. I do not know of any literature which devotes itself to examining the psychological impact of carrier status disclosure.* Certainly, it is an issue that needs much more attention than it has been given in the past. I suspect that screening programs in the near future will involve groups other than blacks and it would be important to have this knowledge so we could have a better awareness of what it means to be labeled a carrier of a genetic trait.

There is nothing I know of, outside of some of the literature I cited in my paper, on carrier status disclosure in genetic counseling. But that should be a little different than disclosure in mass screening, because the former is usually confined to the family. The effects on the family, as I briefly indicated, can be quite devastating.

**Dr. Ferholt:** Is there anybody who would like to respond to the question of the racial implication of the national focus on sickle cell anemia?

**Dr. Hsia:** The answer to that question is partly economic. The cost of testing for some hemoglobinopathies is about $1 per person at present. The chance of finding a carrier for sickle cell hemoglobin is about one in ten if the black population is screened. There are hemoglobin abnormalities which affect non-blacks, but the chance of finding them is much lower, about one in one thousand or less. The differential frequency in population subgroups determines where the most returns can be obtained per unit cost.

---

*See Hampton, M.L., Anderson, J., Lavizzo, B.S., and Bergman, A.B. Sickle cell "non-disease", a potentially serious public health problem. Am. J. Dis. Child. 1974. In press.—Eds.

There is excessive misapprehension about what the intent of the test should be. I think the test should give those people, who are identified as carriers, information that they can choose to use or not use. They have a right to this information. I don't believe that anyone else has a right to use this information to the detriment of those who are identified as carriers. I think there is a serious need for careful studies on the impact of screening programs on all people who are screened as to whether they understand why they are being screened, whether they have agreed to the screening, whether they adequately understand the results of the screening. We are hoping to initiate this kind of study in collaboration with some community groups.

**Dr. Jemison:** Would the expense of testing the entire population be any greater for non-blacks than it is for those of us whose children are tested for PKU? Would the frequency of positives be any greater considering the source of many persons for parents in America?

**Dr. Bender:** I think it would be ideal if every child were screened in this country as completely as possible as part of a routine, thorough physical examination. Perhaps all couples could be screened at the time that they are married, regardless of color.

I think one of the problems is shown in the data that Dr. Hsia presented. The Yale Genetics Clinic looked at 177 people this past year in one of the best programs I have ever heard about. But if they had to look at all the people in New Haven, they could not do it.

At present, there just are not enough geneticists and people capable of doing this and the general public has not been educated to evaluate such information. But I think you are right, it might be ideal if everyone were tested.

**Dr. Hsia:** The blacks are not being discriminated against because they are being screened. They are being offered the benefit of a screening test which as yet is not being offered to everyone who might benefit from it.

**Dr. Ferholt:** I don't want to leave the last word to people on the podium. The question was asked why and by whom it was decided to screen blacks first? Are there some racial implications in that selection? That question still remains. Although these answers are relevant, they do not directly answer the question.

**Mr. Brosseau:** I am George Brosseau from the National Science Foundation. Most of the impetus for sickle cell screening programs comes from the black community. But black communities are divided among themselves as to whether screening is desirable or undesirable. So to some extent there is an intrinsic racial orientation to sickle cell screening. However, the deeper issue arises because screening programs are compulsory in many places. Some laws state, for example, that all black children in first grade must be screened. That is discriminatory. What is more serious is that screening offers no obvious benefit as yet. This is a disease for which there is no treatment and so you are providing people with information that may work to their detriment with no concomitant, demonstrable benefit. A real problem with sickle cell screening is that the cost-benefit equation has not been worked out in a way that shows what is the benefit. Therefore, all we see are the detriments, and the detriments are racially maldistributed. Blacks suffer these detriments much more than whites.

**Dr. Rosenberg:** I would like to disagree with the last statement made by Mr. Brosseau from the National Science Foundation. I do not believe that one can define benefit only in terms of therapy. I think the screening programs for sickle cell trait testing have been started with the idea of trying to prevent the birth of children with sickle cell anemia if the family chooses. I think it is very hard to say that that is a program without benefit.

**Mr. Brosseau:** I think you missed the point. It has not been demonstrated that compulsory screening of first grade children will have any effect on reproductive decisions. If one is concerned about that I think it might be much more helpful to make available a voluntary premarital screening program. The potential of prevention is likely to be much greater that way.

**Retired Statistician:** I don't see why, given the small extra cost of applying or encouraging the screening of all children in places like Washington where a large or substantial proportion is black, all the children should not be screened and accept the extra cost.

**Miss Desmoyers:** I am Ann Desmoyers, Northeastern University. Dr. Bender, I was very outraged by your stand on the ethical issues concerned here. I think if we are going to address the ethical issues, we must be very realistic about what the social situation is in this country. You seemed taken aback by the attitude of some people toward sickle cell anemia — they would like not to be screened. I wonder if you are aware of some of the implications for black people with sickle cell anemia? Did you know for instance, that a black stewardess who has sickle cell trait may not be allowed to fly or may be refused some jobs on this basis? There is also an instance of a truck driver losing his job because he was found to be a carrier. I wonder if you are also familiar with Richard Herrnstein of Harvard University who last year wrote an article he titled, "IQ" in which he suggested that IQ is genetically inherited and that blacks had a lower IQ than whites. In an interview subsequent to that in MIT's *Ergo* he suggested IQ data be taken in the 1980 Census and then used as part of a eugenics program in this country. Also, I thing that the emphasis on sickle cell anemia which we find in the current press is contributing in very large part to a campaign of racism which is sweeping the country, as manifested by the works of such pseudoscientists as Herrnstein, Moynahan, Eysenck, and Jensen. I don't think we should pass over this lightly. There are ethical implications to these abuses and we will see a lot of concrete racist measures as a consequence.

**Dr. Bender:** I was trying to develop the point that there is a prevalent and an ever-growing problem dealing with, for want of a better term, the right not to know. I think that, as scientists and educators, we in part have failed to deal with this particular syndrome.

We have not made it our business to be certain that the public, and public agencies, fully understand complex scientific problems and issues. The result has often been partial understanding or irrational public policy. But, in addition, there are people who wish to play ostrich, who wish to avoid the issues, who wish not to know about such things as the potential deleterious genes that they carry. I am concerned about that. Whether you find that offensive or not, it is true. And I think that this is something that we, as educators, have to grapple with.

**Dr. Hsia:** I think the young lady has every right to be outraged, but she must remember what she is being outraged against. I flew down to this conference. That does not mean I support the use of airplanes for bombing. I think the question of using screening tests to help people know about their genes is quite different from people misusing this information in ignorance or in malicious intent to exercise racism. The point is not solely whether screening is being misused. That is very important, but the point is also whether screening should be used properly and how this can be done.

**Miss Blustein:** I am Bonnie Blustein of Science for People, SDS, University of Pennsylvania. I think when we are talking about the issue of how screening and testing affects black people, we have to see it in the context of how the whole movement towards genetic control is going to affect black people. A historical perspective is useful. A recent symposium on genetics included a specific example of genetic counseling in the 1920's. Many geneticists then, with virtually no opposition, were asserting without adequate scientific basis that children of racially mixed parents have an increased probability of genetic defect. Dr. Hsia started out his presentation by saying we all want our children to be attractive, intelligent, and free from genetic diseases. The last discussor mentioned theories of genetic inferiority of black people. Very prestigious people are putting this forward and getting tremendous publicity, tremendous acclaim. In fact, one example of this is a statement in the *American Psychologist* signed by four Nobel Prize winners and a number of other prestigious people saying there should be more research on the hereditary basis of social behavior.

Most of us are here today in this symposium because we see there is a positive use of genetics in helping people. I think we should be aware that the whole eugenics movement now, like in the 1920's, is ripe to be used for public racism or genocide in this country. I would like to propose that as a symposium, we take a stand condemning the historical role the eugenics movement has played in building and justifying racism.

**Dr. Ferholt:** It is not appropriate or meaningful for us to vote here on any proposals, but we appreciate what you said.

Many speakers are stressing the need to question the basic assumption that it is desirable to make genetic choices at all if we do not have the controls to insure the way those choices are made and to make sure that they remain directed towards ethical and good ends. I think we ought to continue speaking to that issue if we can.

**Dr. Ivker:** I am Frances Ivker from Louisiana State University, New Orleans. I would like to call for greater recognition of the Government's responsibility in sponsoring genetic screening. Consider Tay-Sachs disease. Dr. Kaback pointed out that there was a very positive benefit to be gained. Yet the Government has seemed to be unresponsive to the funding of such a project. Now that we have talked about the positive aspects of genetic screening and counseling for those who want it on a voluntary basis, I would like to call for greater government financial support for such projects. Optimal genetic screening requires public education so that the public can intelligently decide upon the desirability and the financial feasibility of screening for specific conditions. The main emphasis of the symposium should be to bring to the public's and to the Government's attention the need for supporting such programs at this time.

**Mr. Eisenstark:** I am Howard Eisenstark of the Genetics Department at Stanford. Concerning educating the public and the Government about genetic counseling services, I wonder if there was or will be any effort to do something like the Tay-Sachs television commercial or television's VD commercials to educate the public and also if any lobbying may be done to educate legislators about genetic counseling and available services?

**Dr. Ferholt:** This question will be approached more this afternoon in the discussions about implementation of social policy. So let's table it until then.

**A Student:** Dr. Sorenson spoke about the problems with individual genetic counseling to the effect that the major problems seem to be the social stigma attached to the results of the counseling. He remarked that many patients do not want to realize there is a problem or to accept it and many individuals fear the reactions of other people to knowing about the individual's genetic problem. This seems to be a major block in the application of genetic counseling.

I would like to know what is being done to find out why these attitudes exist. That really is an essential part of it because there cannot be the useful application of genetic counseling unless there are solutions to the problems of social stigma, personal denial, and the like.

**Dr. Sorenson:** I would like to say two things in regard to that.

First of all, I think it is important to realize that whereas some studies point up that about 50 percent of the couples experience some type of problem in understanding or accepting genetic counseling, they report at the same time that fully 50 percent do get something out of it and are able to use this knowledge in some fashion.

But looking at those 50 percent that experience some type of a problem, I think such problems have several sources. One is the historical legacy in this country that determines, to some degree, what it means to have a hereditary problem. This legacy is rooted, in part, in the early association of racism with applied genetics in the United States. This major historical legacy adds to the stigmatization of a person or family having a genetic problem.

On the other hand, the current attention being given to screening programs, the light being shed on the nature of genetic problems, and increasing public realization that all of us carry anywhere from 4 to 10 deleterious genes will in some respect start correcting this. People will more readily admit there is a problem in their family and seek competent medical advice.

**A Social Worker:** I am a social worker in Rehabilitation Programs.

I would like to know about cystic fibrosis and how it is transmitted.

**Dr. Hsia:** It is an autosomal recessive disease, with a 25 percent recurrence risk to families who have had at least one affected child. The gene is quite common (one in twenty) among people of Western European extraction.

**A Social Worker:** Would you suggest that a family be counseled if, for instance, a sister of one of the parents has cystic fibrosis? How far back would you suggest counseling?

**Dr. Hsia:** We suggest anyone who is worried about genetic problems should try to find an authority to give them accurate information and resolve their worries.

**Mrs. Silverberg:** Our cystic fibrosis center counsels and gives information about cystic fibrosis offspring. Many do act on it. We are hoping there will be a way of detecting the carrier state of that very common disease. Then our counseling could provide even more information.

**Dr. Ferholt:** I want to point out that several speakers have questioned the attitude of our society, not only to racial deviance, but to deviance in general. Many wonder how the promulgation of the choice of genetic information might affect our attitudes toward deviance and what that may do for individuals in society.

**Dr. Glass:** I am Bentley Glass, State University of New York at Stony Brook. I want to add a further word about this problem of stigmatization. I think the proper answer to be made in genetic counseling to this fear is that all of us, with a very high degree of probability, carry somewhere between 4 and 10 harmful genetic factors. In all humility, I will say that I know of at least three I possess myself. In other words, we are all stigmatized. The problems arise when, because of the choices of marriage mates, two individuals with the same defective genes marry one another. This is a stroke of bad luck that happens not infrequently — with higher probability for some genetic conditions in certain segments of the population than for other conditions. Hence no other segment of the population is to be regarded as stigmatized, and no individual is to be regarded as stigmatized. I think that in our genetic counseling we have to make that very clear.

**Citizen from Redding Ridge:** I am from Redding Ridge, Connecticut. I would like to ask what the cost is of a genetic work-up?

**Dr. Hsia:** There is a big difference between the cost and the charge. We charge $75 for families who can afford it. We charge less for families who can afford less. The cost of various laboratory tests and other things are not included in that figure.

# III. CHOOSING OUR CHILDRENS' GENES: IMPACT ON SOCIETY

# THE MORAL THREAT OF PERSONAL MEDICINE

**Garrett Hardin**

*Department of Biological Sciences, University of California, Santa Barbara*

When we use the word "medicine" we usually mean personal medicine, medicine aimed at alleviating the problems of the individual. Personal medicine seldom considers the needs of society as a whole (which are sometimes not congruent with merely personal needs), and almost never consider the interests of posterity. Unfortunately, practicing personal medicine to relieve the effects of hereditary defects works against the interests of posterity. The justification of this assertion is quite simple.

The mutation process is unstoppable, and most new mutations are harmful. Good mutations are literally as rare as hen's teeth. Under natural conditions, bad mutations are eliminated by the process we call natural selection. The effect of medical measures is to diminish the force of natural selection, thereby increasing the genetic load in the next generation.

## SHORTCOMINGS OF PROSTHETICS

At this point, one might say: "But does this really matter? After all, medicine treats the person by diminishing the phenotypic effects of his genes, whatever they are. If the phenotypic bad effects of genes are diminished why worry about the partially hidden genes themselves? Aren't medical prosthetics just as good as the real thing?"

The answer is *No*, for several reasons. In the first place, almost every prosthetic device has what one might call a "simple" defect. Poor eyesight we remedy with eye glasses; this works pretty well, but just ask anyone who wears glasses if he functions as well as somebody who doesn't. If nothing else, when he gets out in the rain, he wishes his glasses had windshield wipers. That's the sort of thing I mean by a "simple" defect.

More complicated defects are what we might call cybernetic defects — lack of sophistication in design to take care of many different circumstances. For example, crutches (which I can speak about from experience) suffer from the great defect of having no knees. Just try to walk on ice without bending your knees! Of course, we might engineer some knees into the crutches, together with the necessary feedbacks. What would this cost? Ten thousand dollars? Would the result ever be as good as real knees? Effective cybernetic systems are both subtle and expensive, if they have to be made by human art.

Hormone therapy suffers from a similar defect — lack of sophisticated, sensitive feedbacks. Ask anyone who is "on thyroid." It is hard to match ingestion with unpredictable and varying needs which express themselves with a considerable time-delay.

Consider phenylketonuria (PKU). We try to minimize the damage by restricting the intake of phenylalanine. This amino acid is both indispensable and dangerous to PKU youngsters; trying to ingest the right amount is like trying to balance oneself on a knife edge. It is hell for the families that have to monitor the life of a PKU child. There is a regrettable lack of candor in medical reporting of the "successes" of diet control in PKU: the psychological trauma is usually swept under the rug. Think of having a PKU child in the family and having to watch it every moment of the day every day of the year; having (in effect) to be its jailer, having to inhibit all the child's spontaneity in eating. Even if we grant that PKU can be controlled by diet — and it is not completely clear that it can — the resultant anticybernetic life with its attendant psychological stresses is a mighty poor way to live.

The financial cost of prosthetics is often great. There are signs that the public is waking up to this. You have heard that it takes $25,000 a year to keep a Tay-Sachs child alive, for the tragic few years of its existence. I notice a recent news report that the best treatment of hemophiliacs, involving frequent transfusions of the missing factors from the blood of normal people, costs some $22,000 a year. The same report states that there are about 100,000 hemophiliacs in the United States. The studies of Stevenson and Kerr[1] would suggest that 20,000 to 25,000 is a more reasonable estimate. This means giving the best possible treatment to American hemophiliacs would cost about half a billion dollars per year. This is only the directly identifiable medical expenses; and hemophilia is only one of a long list of hereditary diseases.

Prosthetics should never be regarded as a complete substitute for the real thing. They are always second best. And we shouldn't pride ourselves too much on how much we can do with prosthetics. We must not forget the genetic malfunctions that make prosthetics necessary.

## PROSTHETIC THREAT TO POSTERITY

The gravest danger arises when the use of prosthetics in personal medicine increases the number of children produced by the bearers of hereditary defects over what it would be if prosthetics were not used. Personal medicine is then in conflict with community medicine. The increase in genetic load is slow, but it is inexorable if personal medicine is not coupled with some control of breeding.

Perhaps an analogy will help. The reproduction of genetic material has some points of resemblance to the printing of a book. But whereas thousands or even millions of books can be printed from one type-setting, each genetic "setting" is used only for a few replications. The analogy would be closer if the first printing of a book were used as the model to set up type for the second copy, which was used as the model for setting up type for the third copy, and so on. Each replication of the genetic "type" brings a fresh exposure to the risk of making "typographical errors," i.e., mutations.

Under natural conditions, natural selection is the proofreader that eliminates "typographical errors". Whenever our humanitarian impulses lead us to employ personal medicine to protect individuals against the proofreader the ultimate effect of our good intentions is to increase the number of errors as the mutation process continues to add new errors to the old ones already protected. In the genetic process, errors are copied just as faithfully as correct readings. Of course a second error at the same place in the text *might* correct the first, but probability is against it. (Who would rely on the unguided carelessness of typesetters to correct a text rich in "typos"?)

## HEROIC TREATMENT A RIGHT?

Let's return to the problem of hemophilia with its potential societal cost of half a billion dollars a year. Just recently four hemophiliacs have brought a class action suit in one of the eastern Federal courts to compel the U.S. Department of Health, Education and Welfare to give the best medical treatment known free to all hemophiliacs in the United States. The plaintiffs argue that such treatment is a human *right*. Since the "best treatment" would require a generosity in the giving of blood by normal people that may not exist it is likely that the hemophiliacs' demand cannot be met in any case. But (for the sake of argument) let us put this objection aside and ask if the demand is the sort that society *should* accede to? Half a billion dollars is a lot of money; and hemophilia is only the tip of the iceberg of hereditary defects.

For the courts to establish a new right to the best personal medicine for all citizens, for all diseases, would be to establish a devastating drain on the economy of the country — which would adversely affect the welfare of all citizens, whatever their genetic constitution. I await the decision of the court with trepidation.

## GENETIC RESPONSIBILITY

One way to look at problems like this is in terms of that much abused word *responsibility*. We must admit that if there is one thing a person is not responsible for, it is the genes that were passed on to him. No one has the opportunity to pick his parents. One can sympathize with hemophiliacs and, indeed, with the bearers of all hereditary genetic errors. But that is literally *each* of us, as Bentley Glass has pointed out: every one of us bears (in all probability) at least one hereditary error, great or small — and these errors were not of our choosing. We are not responsible as the recipients of errors.

But should we not be responsible as the transmitters of errors? If there are some people in society who refuse to take such responsibility, who say *No* for whatever reason, refusing to inhibit their own breeding in spite of the fact they are passing on genes known to be undesirable genes, does not then the issue of responsibility arise in a very acute form? Consider the case of a hemophiliac (almost invariably a male). His children, with rare exceptions, will all be asymptomatic. But his daughters will have one dose of the gene. When it comes time for them to reproduce, half of the sons of the daughters will (on the average) be hemophiliacs. With a delay of one generation the hemophiliac who insists on reproducing is saddling posterity with his problem.

Should individual freedom extend so far? Should individual freedom include the freedom to impose upon society costs that society does not want? This is the issue all of us must face. When such costs are very slight, we might avoid the issue by saying that the law is not concerned with trifles. But hemophilia, Tay-Sachs, sickle cell anemia and PKU are not trifles.

We must recognize that this is a finite world. The money we spend for one purpose, we cannot spend on another. If we spend all our income on the phenotypic correction of genetic defects there will be very little left for preserving an adequate quality of life.

This is one of mankind's major problems. It doesn't require an immediate solution; but let us keep the issues clearly in mind so that we do not

lightly assert such a thing as a right to breed under any and all circumstances, regardless of the consequences.

## ENVY AND EUGENICS

What I have been discussing, of course, is eugenics. The practice of
eugenics is often divided into two classes; negative and positive. By negative
eugenics, we mean the taking of such measures as will diminish the genetic
load in later generations. By positive eugenics, we mean taking measures
that might in a positive way improve the quality of human life for future
generations. We can do this by encouraging the breeding of people who are
unusually low in genetic defects, and perhaps unusually well-endowed with
desirable human "talents."

In all of the years of its very checkered career, eugenics has had its only
successes (and they haven't been many) in gaining the assent of society to
the practice of negative eugenics. The reason for this, I think, is quite clear:
negative eugenics is the only form that is easily reconcilable with the
universal human phenomenon of *envy*.[2]

Each of us can comparatively easily agree to the institution of negative
eugenic measures because he can say to himself: "Well, *I* am essentially
O.K.,; as for this small minority of *other* people who aren't O.K., I am
perfectly willing to admit they are my inferiors, so I will accept in-
fringements of their liberty. Negative eugenics doesn't threaten *me*."

Positive eugenics is another matter. To single out a few people as being
unusually superior and seeing to it they have more children than the average
does threaten me because I will probably be left out of this select group.
Envious, I will say, "How come they are better than I am?" or I might try to
base my objection on general principles: "We should never make invidious
comparisons."

The adjective "invidious," I would remind you, is derived from the
Latin word for envy. It means provoking envy. Because of envy, positive
eugenic measures are not, I think, a possibility for the near future. The most
we can hope for, for a long time, is negative eugenics.

## ETHICS AND THE TIMING OF SELECTION

The cost of negative eugenics is dependent upon the stage at which we
employ selection. Should we eliminate unsatisfactory gametes; or unsatisfactory embryos; or unsatisfactory newborn babies; or unsatisfactory

adults? Clearly, without making any large argument here, we should be able to agree that the earlier the stage at which we make the elimination, the more acceptable it is for everybody. The purpose of prenatal diagnosis is to identify defective individuals before they are born, while the cost of selection is *comparatively* little. We are less unwilling to sacrifice embryos than we are to sacrifice newborn children.

As far as the genetic effect is concerned, it is precisely the same whether we sacrifice a gamete, an embryo, a newborn child or an adult before reproduction.* The eugenic effect is exactly the same. But the human costs, in terms of both ordinary economic costs and the more subtle emotional costs, are clearly less the earlier the sacrifice is made. So the aim of eugenics is to identify a defect at the earliest possible stage so as to eliminate it before the individual and society have made any appreciable investment in the unwanted genotype.

In this connection, I take issue with one of the earlier participants who spoke hopefully of the fact that we might some day be able to operate surgically upon embryos *in utero*. This seems to me to be an unwise goal, because such surgery would surely be exceedingly expensive and exceedingly difficult under the best of circumstances. Let me be blunt. In terms of both money and emotions an early embryo (say a 12-weeks fetus) has had so little invested in it that the loss from aborting it will certainly be much less than the financial cost of heroic fetal surgery, and (I expect) less than the emotional cost to the parents anxiously awaiting the outcome for another 28 weeks. I frankly think that the goal of fetal surgery serves principally the ego needs of surgeons and is destructive of the even more valid ego needs of parents. My heart is with the parents. Fortunately, that is where the interests of economics and eugenics lie also.

---

*In the simple sense that the non-reproducing individual does not directly contribute to the gene pool. Such a person might have other genetic effects. — Eds.

## References

1.  STEVENSON, A.C., and KERR, C.B. On the distribution of frequencies of mutation to genes determining harmful traits in man. *Mutation Res. 4*:339-352, 1967.

2.  SCHOECK, H. *Envy.* Harcourt, Brace and World, New York, 1966.

3.  HARDIN, G. The tragedy of the commons. *Science 162*:1243-1248, 1968.

# GENETICS, CHOICE AND SOCIETY

## John Fletcher

*Director, Interfaith Metropolitan Theological Education, Inc., 1419 V. Street N.W. Washington, D.C.*

I have been asked by the organizers of the panel to estimate some of the long-term effects of genetic proposals on society while paying particular attention to the welfare and rights of individuals. Accepting this task thrust me into the midst of the tensions between the claims of society and the claims of individual rights.

When I am honest, I must state that I am in considerable conflict about the morality of futuristic techniques like *in vitro* fertilization or extrauterine gestation. I can respond to the desire of a woman with blocked oviducts for *in vitro* fertilization of her ovum by her husband's sperm for re-implantation into her uterus. But there is something in my blood which resists the growth of fetuses apart from families or apart from mothers who delegate them to surrogate mothers.

Perhaps I could be persuaded if I could see more consequences that would be beneficial to such people. But as of today, I am in considerable moral doubt about the benefits of surrogate parents and prenatal adoption.

## GENETICS AND SOCIAL CHANGES

The scientific and moral literature of the past few years shows that my conflict is widespread. For several months I have been a member of a task force investigating these issues.[1] In this role I have learned that current genetic interventions like screening and counseling create and exacerbate conflict. Therefore, to think about more futuristic proposals such as those under discussion here is to complicate and compound the conflict almost beyond tolerance. The prospect of deliberate genetic intervention evokes the deepest level of belief about good and evil and about the being and destiny of mankind. As a member of interdisciplinary task forces during the past four years, I have observed and read more concentrated theological and philosophical discussion between scientists and their colleagues from other disciplines than I have among theologians.

The basic social conflict in applied genetics stems, on the one hand, from the need to change ourselves, to change our condition, to enlarge our options, to release ourselves from arbitrariness and, on the other hand, from the need to respect our limits and especially to restrain our tendency towards injustice.

The problem posed by applied genetics is very complicated because of the degree to which it would promise to expand power and freedom and shift well-known limits and the perception of limits. I do not find it unusual that we are in conflict about this topic. Change is conflict, and rapid change is a constant characteristic of our society.

Society is not one thing. At times Dr. Hardin argues as if society were one thing. Society embraces many conflicting interests and groups. Society does not set goals, for society has no mind or personality. To be more accurate, representatives of specific groups help to set goals which are always to some degree in conflict with the goals of other groups. Certain potent and powerful individuals have much to do with the way goals are perceived and set. Thus, society is a conflict which cools off occasionally to allow for indispensable ceremonies of goal-setting, vision-making, and conflict resolution.

My attitude about estimating effects of genetic programs on society is that even such estimating is risky since we here today help or hinder applied genetics. But non-scientists must make this effort or else leave the task of estimating effects entirely to scientists thereby abdicating their responsibilities for nurturing values and challenging the *status quo*.

In making estimates our starting point should be what we know about ourselves and our values rather than a projected ideal "knowledge" of what we might be in the future. And here I differ from a scientist like Robert Sinsheimer who makes eloquent arguments about the future of genetics.[2] I am a subscriber to ideas of ethical realism in most matters and especially in this one. The human enterprise is too hopeful to justify ethical pessimism, and it is too tragic to justify ethical optimism. We need an ethic which at once releases our hope and restrains our injustice. The "predictions" which follow are propositions or hypotheses based upon an attempt to be ethically realistic.

## SOCIETY, THE INDIVIDUAL, AND THE FUTURE
## OF GENETICS

First, there will be more and not less disagreement about the wisdom of trying to "control" human evolution in either a biological or a cultural sense. There is no way to control human evolution without seriously interfering with the destinies of individuals and groups.

There will be less disagreement about organizing systematic attacks on certain catastrophic and some less than catastrophic genetic diseases, but even these must be mounted with the utmost sensitivity to the real political and social relationships of the groups involved.

As the history of the screening for sickle cell disease and its carrier state already shows, it is no simple matter to speak of "control" of that disease or its carriers. The first spate of laws, state and municipal, referring to sickle cell screening tend to be riddled with medical and racial mythology and fail to assist leaders in black communities to educate, screen, and counsel. For example, in an effort to screen pre-maritally for sickle hemoglobin, the legislature of New York State stated, "such test as may be necessary shall be given to each applicant for a marriage license who is not of the Caucasian, Indian or Oriental race for the purposes of discovering the existence of sickle cell anemia."[3] This extraordinary statement obscures the fact that others than blacks may carry the trait and have sickle cell anemia. The omission speaks loudly of racial obfuscation. Another important example occurred when the District of Columbia declared sickle cell anemia a communicable disease.[4] The term "communicable" in ordinary language means something quite different from an inherited genetic condition.

Biological progress will uncover more possibilities for control, but the resistance to being controlled will rise proportionately.

Second, because new genetic proposals belong to the category of human experimentation and because the tradition of voluntarism essentially controls the relations between patient and physician in Western culture, there is no real possibility of mounting a widespread program of mandatory positive eugenics without displacing this voluntarism. Massive mandatory conscription of persons for medical experiments works against voluntarism. Displacement of voluntarism would erase any perception of benefits from positive eugenics.

Third, there will be a growing emphasis upon applying knowledge about genetic disease and carrier states to decision-making regarding marriage and childbearing. There will be a slowly growing effort to avoid serious genetic mishaps which can be detected prior to birth.

There should not be a social policy which approves a long-range strategy of abortion of genetically defective fetuses following prenatal diagnosis as a substitute for developing genetic therapies. The healing and not the elimination of handicapped human life should be our goal.

It is wrong to designate abortion of a defective fetus as "therapy." Therapy implies that one is curing a disease.* Abortion is, quite clearly, a form of killing a premature and defective life. A fetus is not a "person" in the conscious, fully developed sense. But a fetus is an early human form of life on the way to being a person.

I believe that the arguments used by Dr. Hardin and Dr. Schelling promoting abortion are deficient in that they promote reliance upon sanction by the state for justification of abortion. At this stage of the development of genetic medicine, the parent-child bond will be stable only if parents are able to tell children, tested or untested, "We made the decision to enter testing because of specific and known risks and we made the decision." The more personal and the less coerced a decision, the more opportunity for personally telling children the reasons for it. Dr. Schelling argues precisely the opposite, but I cannot fathom how a child can feel more confidence in a father who tells him that he had to have prenatal diagnosis (and thus contemplate his child's destruction) because the state commanded it, than he would have in a father who took personal responsibility for that decision. Nothing could weaken or dissolve the parent-child bond more effectively than children becoming afraid that their parents made such decisions for trivial reasons of personal convenience or because they were forced into it for external societal reasons.

Only parents who are definitely at risk for genetically defective children should be offered amniocentesis. The risks of the procedure justify this stricture, and the ethics of parenthood do so even more. Prevention of known and verifiable risk of serious genetic disease may, in particular families, be acceptable to protect the family. Some families cannot survive the addition of one more defective child. I do not propose this as a general principle for all families. In other families it is not *inevitable* that the severely handicapped person can expect little or no fulfillment in life. The only warrant, at present, which justifies abortion following prenatal diagnosis is the combination of a

---

*As Kaback describes, the dis-ease here may be the parents' fear of conceiving a defective child—Eds.

positive diagnosis and the projection of undue hardship or misery for a particular family. Both factors must be taken into account in making a decision, or else the prospective abortion will have been considered without weighing the impact on the specific family.

The application of genetic knowledge to man must be kept within the framework of the ultimate goal of medicine, to heal the sick individual or family of disease. Therapy is the goal. We should not become accustomed to abortion of illness or confuse that with therapy.

Mass genetic screening similarly should not be mandatory because of the climate of threat which mandatory genetic intervention introduces into a flexible and pluralistic society. At least on a scale from mandatory to voluntary, there should never be mandatory screening where there is no therapy.

Four, suppose one takes amniocentesis and prenatal diagnosis to be the first major intervention due to genetic knowledge in family life. In an exploratory study with 25 couples, I developed a hypothesis that prenatal diagnosis does not decrease affection of parents for tested children.[5]

I conducted four interviews with couples who were at risk for genetically defective children and who requested amniocentesis: prior to genetic counseling, prior to the test, following the test, and following abortion or the birth of the child. My findings substantiated the basic hypothesis. These parents felt "closer" to their tested children. However, considerable moral suffering was involved in making the decision to request amniocentesis. Wanting children desperately, yet having to contemplate the possible abortion of a defective fetus, these parents were often torn asunder with worry. The most acute time was in the interim following amniocentesis and prior to the results. From this exploratory study I developed several hypotheses for further research:

1.  Consideration of abortion is the major moral problem of parents in genetic counseling.

2.  Parents are inclined to favor abortion in case of a positive diagnosis, and they have reached this position prior to counseling.

3.  Parents in genetic counseling do not favor abortion "on demand" but only for specific, medically indicated reasons.

4.  Parents feel morally competent to make decisions in genetic counseling without seeking non-medical advice.

5.  More moral suffering occurs when parents are faced with choices including sterilization as well as abortion.

6.  The counselor's wishes for outcomes in a case will be conveyed directly or indirectly to the patient.

7.  Although Catholic mothers are more ready to accept a genetically defective child, there will be more Catholics seeking prenatal diagnosis due to the autonomy (from the Church) of the family in issues of reproduction.

Follow-up studies of parents one year or more following amniocentesis and negative diagnosis, showed some ambivalence about the effects of amniocentesis on the parent-child relationship, since parents were still perplexed about having contemplated the abortion of their living child.[6] But on the whole, there was a quite positive reaction. Every couple stated that amniocentesis took the terror out of childbearing when there was genetic risk involved. Some parents said that they knew their tested children longer than they had known their untested children. They gave them names in the third or fourth month. They even prepared their rooms accordingly and bought blue or pink clothes. One could speculate that prenatal genetic information can deepen the sense of intimacy between parent and child as it hastens and increases the assumption of parenthood before birth.

Genetic knowledge should over the long run improve the chances of stable marriages between carriers. It is well known that a genetically defective child provokes a sense of guilt or doom in the parents. By the same token contemplate the effects of mandatory prenatal diagnosis or mandatory abortion for carrier parents or at-risk groups. One might suppose that because there was less personal responsibility involved with contemplating the possible abortion of one's own child, there would be more of a climate of threat to parent-child relationships from society's mandate and hence less affection and intimacy between parent and child.

I see nothing in the promise of the application of genetic knowledge which will automatically raise us to a higher state of development in the history of evolution. Mankind will not be saved from destruction by genetic knowledge, but neither will we be dehumanized by its careful and restrained use. What we must speak out against is the hasty and often biased way genetic experimentation may be used before preliminary animal or human studies have been done or the too hasty translation of genetic knowledge into laws which further depress and debase minority groups.

My own bias is that the goals toward which genetic science moves should be focused indirectly, if at all, on projects of social or cultural improvement such as the alleviation of aggression, the perpetuation of certain genotypes or the prenatal stimulation of intelligence. My reason for this evolves around the concept of consent which is not only a touchstone of medical ethics, but the cornerstone of political ethics. Since genetic experimentation is irreversible, the more grandiose plans for positive eugenics would not be ethical. Under present conditions, if our generation or the next deliberately decided to experiment on another generation without its consent, this would constitute an irreversible act of aggression against a future generation. Yet, we must not be frightened into putting a freeze on the application of genetic knowledge to disease. We must restrain our power to change the next generation, but we must not restrain our need to be merciful or to heal.

I do not subscribe to the view that a technological society is progressively dehumanizing us. Man makes culture and has the initiative in the culture-making process; the roots of dehumanization lie deeper in us than feedback from technique or technology. There is no ultimate threat to the concept of the sanctity of human life or of the individual from genetic knowledge. Man is an ultimate threat to himself when he is unwilling to accept the anxiety of living in the constantly shifting territory between learning to use his freedom and learning to respect his limits. The anxiety we feel, when we approach such problems bearing such meager wisdom, is a signal that we are in touch with the basic human condition. And this will not change.

# References

1. Task Force on Genetic Screening and Genetic Counseling of the Institute for Ethics, Society and the Life Sciences, Hastings, New York.

2. SINSHEIMER, R.L. Prospects for future scientific developments: Ambush or opportunity, in *Ethical Issues in Human Genetics* (Hilton, B., Callahan, D., Harris, M., Condliffe, P., Berkley, B. editors)., New York Plenum Press, pp. 341-352, 1973.

3. New York State, Chapter 994, Section 13, Sessim Law 1972.

4. Regulation No. 72-9. District of Columbia City Council, May 3, 1972.

5. FLETCHER, J. Parents in Genetic Counseling: The Moral Shape of Decision-Making, (in Hilton *et al., op. cit.*), pp. 301-328.

6. FLETCHER, J. The brink: The parent-child bond in the genetic revolution, *Theological Studies, 33*: 457-485, 1972.

# CHOOSING OUR CHILDREN'S GENES

Thomas C. Schelling

*Professor of Economics, Harvard University*

This week is an interesting time to discuss our subject: newspaper stories of cannibalism in the Andes invite the question regarding what difference there is between eating a dead person's flesh and putting his heart in your chest or his lenses in your eyes.

## CHOOSING OUR WORDS

An earlier writer, commenting on a proposal, wrote that there was "something in his blood" that resisted it. Blood is a favorite metaphor, and the choice of language affects the way we approach these matters. A clone can be anything from a lovable twin to an artifact, according to what image somebody puts in your mind before you even know what he is going to talk about. Word pictures like "gene pool" fix attention on a regularly shaped pool of uniform consistency, and divert attention from interconnected irregular pools with streams and eddies and backwaters.

## CHOOSING OUR CHILDREN'S GENES

Today's title, *Choosing Our Children's Genes*, allows several interpretations. Usually it means all of us, collectively, choosing the genes of the next generation. They are all *our children*, whether or not individually we are parents. Your children and mine are *our children* together in this interpretation — even bachelors can join in calling them *our children*. (The title could even refer to traditional eugenics or animal husbandry, in which the process is one of "choosing our children's parents".) *Choosing*, too, is ambiguous until we identify the menu from which we can select.

I am going to take a literal interpretation of the title *Choosing Our Children's Genes* not because it represents the most impending issue but because it is one issue that interests me. I am going to talk about each of us choosing *his own* children's genes not determining genetic policy for other people and their children. I am furthermore going to discuss choosing genes for children who are literally and biologically *our* children — not choosing genes from a donor, not manufacturing genes.

If my wife and I, or your mate and you, could choose from the available genetic menu a particular inheritance — for me of my child, for you of your child — what choices might be available? What choices might we be motivated to make? And what differences might it make to anybody exactly which choices we made?

## THE MENU OF CHOICE

When two people get together to have a child the number of genetically different children they could have is a large one. The particular child they have is randomly selected, according to current theory, from among a number of potential children that is more than ten thousand times the population of the earth. This is about how many chromosomally different children a couple could have — leaving aside the intrachromosomal differences that arise naturally or that might be engineered.

There are about eight million genetically distinct sperm that I can produce and eight million distinct eggs that my wife might have produced, although she cannot produce anything like that number of eggs. If you multiply those numbers together, you get the number of potentially different children, any one of which we might have conceived. I am going to talk about some of the issues that would arise if I could exercise some choice among those sixty trillion genetically different children, and what I might like to choose.

Despite the large number, this choice is narrowly limited. It is limited to the genetic material that my wife and I possess. We probably cannot have a child as tall as Kareem Jabbar or as musical as Bach, or even a child that looks much like someone selected at random from the audience. We are limited to a number of twofold choices from a limited packet of information that I contain. We are stuck with an even more limited assortment of messages that my wife contains.

So while there are — what did I say? — sixty trillion possible different children we might have, the actual number to select them from may be only a few tens of millions. Like it or not, most of them are going to look like my wife and me. They are not going to depart radically from the types of people that my wife's parents, grandparents and great-grandparents, and mine were.

Notice that within this choice every child is a *natural* child. Any child that we might select by intervening in the process of choosing our chromosomes — eliminating the lottery and making it a matter of choice —

is a child whose *a priori* likelihood of being born to us is about the same as for every other potential child we might have had. There is nothing artificial, nothing manufactured. There is no reason why any child that we might choose couldn't have been the child we had.

Among the eight million or so genetically distinct sperm that I can produce, not only do they all resemble my own inheritance but they come in a limited number of packages. I am supposing that we cannot break open the chromosomes and select genes but are limited to whole chromosomes. If it turns out that you get the musical talent of a paternal grandmother only with bad eyesight, you have to make a choice. If the traits are combined within the same package, or if they are combined within some complementary and interacting packages, you cannot pick and choose gene by gene; you might pick and choose chromosome by chromosome. Now the question is, what kinds of choices might we make?

## THE TECHNOLOGY OF SELECTION

Because we are severely limited in time I shall skip — and I am sure that some of you will think I am cheating — the technology of how this may someday be done. To state it briefly: one has to identify which chromosome of the two, among any one of the pairs we are interested in, a fetus has or a sperm or egg possesses. One then has to identify the characteristics that are determined by that chromosome. (That may not be directly observable). The characteristics then may have to be traced through the ancestors of the individual. Then there has to be a selection or rejection. The object of selection would be either fetus or sperm. (If it should be possible to screen sperm and eggs, there might be a very limited menu of eggs, depending on how many the technology makes available at any time for examination and activation, and a large menu of sperm; the choice would then be exercised much more on the male side of the family than on the female side).

The energy required to examine a single cell and to determine which chromosome it contains may be enough energy to threaten the cell. There would then be no safe way to screen sperm and eggs, only fetuses. That means a *very* limited choice. One will not search among millions of sperm, but look at one fetus at a time and decide whether it is worthwhile to stop and try again.

Whether or not it will appear worthwhile will likely depend on whether we are limited to something like amniocentesis, which seems, even if effective, not to be entirely safe before about three months, or instead will have techniques for obtaining fetal cellular material earlier in pregnancy without harming the fetus.

One example we have — to prove that this is not an empty category of choice — is that it is now medically feasible to ascertain the sex of a fetus and to abort it if the parents don't want that sex. There are other chromosomal characteristics that can be identified, some of which are reported elsewhere in this volume. Those that receive the most attention at present are related to some pathology.

## THE DIRECT COSTS OF SELECTION

At present it is a costly choice at best. The fetus must be carried for about three months and carried without too close a sense of parental identification so that a choice could actually be made to discard it and start over. Starting over, one loses a likely minimum of six months between pregnancies, and it surely costs anxiety and loss of enjoyment of the early months of pregnancy — enjoyment both for parents and possible siblings. So it is by no means "inexpensive" to abort and start over. But it can be done.

If it turns out that cellular material can be obtained and diagnosis performed within a week or two of conception, the choice may become nearly costless — just a matter of which month one decides to let oneself become pregnant according to the sex or other selected characteristics of the child.

## PECULIARITIES OF THE SEX CHOICE

Choice of sex is different from most other choices. People are presently at liberty to express wishes for a boy or a girl. It may be hard for my wife to talk about whether she would not like somebody quite as short as I and whether she wished her own musical talent rather than my lack of it to be inherited in the children. We may find it difficult to discuss whether any ethnic characteristics that she or I have would look nice in our children be they boys or girls. But it is not improper to discuss — and indeed people of all ages and generations do discuss — whether they would like to have a boy or a girl. So there is a legitimacy to that choice that other choices may not yet have. (The legitimacy may be dependent on the belief that there is no real choice — that no *decision* is at stake — and it is all idle conversation!)

But because that choice is feasible, it may induce the kind of technology — it may cover, so to speak, the social overhead costs of developing the technology — by which one can begin to select for chromosomes other than the one that determines the sex of the child.

There may also come with choosing the sex of children some experience, both demographic and intrafamilial experience, with what happens when people intervene in what used to be God's choice or, to use a second metaphor, used to be a choice that God washed her hands of and left to chance.

It is probably important, too, that many characteristics that people might choose for their children depend on the sex of the child. An example is body size. My impression is that many people would deplore a boy that is too small but would not so much deplore a girl who is small and might equally deplore a girl that is "too large" but not so a boy. Inasmuch, therefore, as many of the things that people might choose, if they could choose, would depend on the sex of the child, the sex choice is in many ways an important entry into the subject.

## OTHER CHARACTERISTICS FOR SELECTION

I shall omit discussion of the sex choice itself and get on to some other characteristics. Might you want to consider.

| | |
|---|---|
| Body size? | Eyesight? |
| Longevity? | Athletic ability? |
| Ethnic identity? | IQ? |
| Left- or right-handedness? | Baldheadedness? |

The technology of choice may differ importantly for these different characteristics. Some characteristics relate to continuous variables, like longevity or body size, others to discrete characteristics like left-handedness or perhaps baldness. Some of the discrete choices, like certain "pathologies" may involve screening for an identifiable unique characteristic. Other choices will involve choosing an extreme or average value along a scale. Some choices may be uniquely identified with a particular chromosome. Others may tend to link in a single chromosome but not exclusively. The determinants of some may be distributed among several chromosomes. Physiognomy, for example, may tend to cluster more than, say, longevity. Finally, two or more important characteristics may tend to be largely determined by the same chromosome, making it hard to choose these characteristics independently.

## SOME DEMOGRAPHIC CONSEQUENCES
## OF CHOICE

If most parents for several generations tried to have children just a little larger than most other people, we'd eventually get rather big — "we" being the human race, not we twentieth-century parents. And what the world is going to need in the future is smaller people, not larger ones. Even if you decide you are not much interested in body size, and merely want your child not below the lower decile, and if everybody makes *that* choice, there will be significant effect on average body size. Even the expectation that other parents are going to be selecting somewhat taller children could make parents who would otherwise be willing to take potluck hedge a little in anticipation and avoid children who would have been but moderately short in the parents' generation but might be noticeably below average in their own generation. The result could be analogous to somewhat more familiar kinds of "inflation".

## SOME CULTURAL CONSEQUENCES
## OF SELECTION

If most of you do not much care whether your child is right or left handed but, given a choice, slightly prefer she not be left-handed in case it becomes unfashionable, and if it is easy to choose right-handedness, you may participate in converting left-handedness from a common, innocuous characteristic — even a proud one — to one so rare, that, in order not to inflict that kind of rarity on a child, people would avoid it. A normal characteristic would thus become a "pathology," a stigma, through a myriad of uncoordinated individual choices.

## PREDICTION AS GUESSWORK

This is necessarily a conjectural essay. Whatever our uncertainty about development of the technology and about the chromosomal choices that the technology may discover, there is at least as much uncertainty — not a lack of ingredients for conjecture but a profusion of casual data good for nothing but conjecture — about the choices that people might elect to make, about the expectations people would have about other people's choices and any inducements that would arise from those expectations, about the attitudes and professional advice that would be brought to bear on personal decisions or about the policies that governmental and religious bodies might promote, and about the ways that decisions might be made — decisions that would usually involve a minimum of two persons, the parents, and often more.

It is even difficult to guess which choices might seem deadly serious and which frivolous when the time came. I imagine that the bottom item on my list, baldheadedness, will appear frivolous. Perusal of advertisements suggests that it is an almost, but not quite, innocuous "abnormality". Exploratory speculation about social processes, like choosing characteristics of one's children, sometimes gains a little freedom by focusing on choices that are not too serious. Baldheadedness may be an example of a culturally determined "esthetic" choice that can serve as a proxy for "looks" or "beauty", that might be highly responsive to the frequency rate within the population and that is correlated with sex. It may be illustrative of how discrimination and stigmata are generated in a culture.*

## THE CONTRAST WITH TRADITIONAL EUGENICS

Baldheadedness is furthermore illustrative of a striking difference between the older-fashioned eugenics and the futuristic possibility of chromosomal selection. The difference is this: eugenics, like animal husbandry, selects *parents*. What we are now discussing is the selection of particular chromosomes from the parents. Traditional eugenics — by "traditional eugenics" I mean almost any program that might have been proposed for "choosing our children's genes" a generation ago — involved a yes-no decision whether or not a person should be a parent. (This was not true in animal husbandry because the offspring could be selectively destroyed, sterilized, or prevented from further breeding). It therefore involved interference in one of the most personal rights that a person could claim.

Chromosomal selection of the kind discussed now is more benign. It could be opportunistic, and it could be at the choice of the parents. A "dominant" trait of one parent could be screened out with about a fifty-fifty chance of success. And if sperm could be screened a dominant trait could be selected out of an abundant population of sperm at no cost to the father, except to the extent that the trait selected out may involve a chromosome that one would have preferred on other grounds like sex of the child. Recessive traits located in chromosomes that carry a "signature" that can be identified with particular ancestors could similarly be avoided. With respect to serious pathologies the liberation from a choice between grave risk and

---

*It may also have selective (survival hence reproductive) significance for fair skinned persons in sunny climates — Eds.

childlessness would be enormous — and in some cases already is. The principle applies to the frivolous as well.

Probably the most important constraint is that some characteristics may be determined by the chromosome that determines the sex of the child; this is a good example of linkage within the chromosome. It is also a good example of the special, if not unique, significance of the choice of sex. If a couple wants a boy, or a girl, it is restricted to the characteristics determined by the chromosome that determines sex. But, then, it may also turn out that nearsightedness and musical talent are determined by a single chromosome. Parents who want to choose the genes of their children will have a constrained choice, not a free choice. But it is their choice.

## SOME MOTIVATIONAL AND DEMOGRAPHIC CONFIGURATIONS

The motives for choosing particular traits or measures can be quite diverse. Some traits may be objects of avoidance because they are painful or awkward or fearsome irrespective of their frequency in the population or their cultural status; these would be the unconditional pathologies. Then there may be traits that are dangerous or disagreeable primarily because they are rare or represent extreme values on a distribution; some of these, but not all of them, are disagreeable because they are socially stigmatized. (A few traits may be valuable precisely because they are rare; they may even have economic value because of scarcity.) An important distinction is between the traits one would choose, or the value along some scale that one would choose, independently of the frequencies and averages of the relevant surrounding population, and the choices that are substantially conditioned by one's human environment. Preferred body size must be substantially conditioned: one wants to see over the top of the grass but, if the whole population could be scaled accordingly, it takes a while to decide whether one would rather be three feet tall or six. Some but not all of this conditioning by the human surroundings is competitive: one wants to be about normal size to find clothes and chairs and stair risers and doorknob heights that one can accommodate comfortably, but one also may prefer to be a little larger or a little stronger or a little taller than others because of some advantage. In the competitive cases one presumably confers a disadvantage on others by successfully achieving the advantage of being larger than they; in contrast, musical talent may be something that one tends to enjoy in the surrounding population, and having a musically talented child may benefit his associates more than it puts them to disadvantage.

But the conditioned choices can be to conform or to disperse or to identify, not merely to "fit" or to "excel". One might, for example, want a child to be average in complexion, different in hair color, taller than average, like or unlike one's ethnic group, long-lived but not precocious in development.

These different kinds of preferences could produce quite different dynamic trends. Longevity, if it does not come at the expense of some other desirable characteristic, is likely to be highly valued, especially if it amounts to the avoidance of short-livedness. The non-natural selection exercised by parents in behalf of their children could increase the mean life span by working on some part or all of the frequency distribution. The prospect of longer-lived spouses and companions might make a long life appear even more worthwhile.

It is harder to guess what would happen to facial and other visible ethnic characteristics. Individual choices might bring about either ethnic blending or ethnic differentiation.

IQ might be treated as a competitive trait. Valuable as it may be for its own sake, it may be construed particularly valuable in a competitive society, whether the competition is based on IQ measurements themselves, on the school success to which IQ may contribute, or on competitive success in one's career. If it were widely believed that the genetic mixtures within most parents made it possible by chromosomal selection to raise the expected IQ of a child by many points above what it would have been by chance selection of the chromosomes and if it became widely believed in certain social classes that nearly everybody was taking advantage of this opportunity, parents might feel coerced into practicing selection, not out of any dissatisfaction with the prospective intelligence of their children, but to keep up with the new generation.

## CHOOSING FOR WHOM?

An interesting difference between longevity and IQ is that IQ may focus attention on the *child* that one's baby will become and longevity on the *adult* it will be eventually. If longevity is determined by chromosomes unrelated to IQ, the hardness of choice will depend on whether one is picking an optimal combination of IQ and longevity from among millions of sperm or instead considering abortion of a fetus on the basis of its prospective IQ and longevity. The parents, who are about to have a baby, probably think more about the child it will be than about the old man or woman it will eventually be.

At the same time, these parents are not themselves children. The father may not expect to have a baldheaded schoolboy, but if he's old enough to do a little estate planning at the prospect of an enlarged family he may be thinking of *his* life and what he would wish for himself if he could wish for the things he is about to choose for his child.

## SOME CONSEQUENCES OF
## HAVING A CHOICE

There are at least two respects in which an ability to choose chromosomes might be unwelcome. One is that some of the things that we might be most motivated to choose have the quality that if we all choose what we individually prefer we are all a little worse off. The illustration I have used is body size; it may be an advantage to be a little larger than others, it is no collective advantage to have the average height and body size move up. Some minor nuisances could become stigmata if they became less common, without disappearing altogether, through a massive "unpopularity contest." A few examples are no proof that the collective social and demographic consequences would outweigh the gains. But the examples remind us that there is nothing about externally conditioned, voluntary choices that guarantees they lead to any collective benefit.

The other difficulty is within the family itself. An example is the choice of the sex of the baby. This is one more thing for the prospective parents to be in disagreement about, with each other and with the grandparents. (If the technique of choice is at all unsure, they run the risk of getting a girl or a boy after together committing themselves to a preference for a boy or a girl). The family that already has a boy and a girl and plans on one more may be almost in the position of delivering a "verdict", in the presence of two children, after trying one of each.

The skinny boy whose mother insists on violin lessons may wonder whether "he" might not have been big like the other boys if his mother hadn't traded size for musical talent before he was old enough to be asked what he preferred. And he may not be satisfied with the answer that "he" comes in only one size: the alternative was some other little boy or girl from among those sixty trillion.

# ETHICAL ISSUES IN GENETIC CHOICES

### Roger L. Shinn

*Union Theological Seminary*

My intention is to think about some of the more ambitious genetic programs that have been seriously proposed. If you ask why I am crossing bridges and thinking about crossing them before we get to them, I have two reasons.

One is that I believe mankind has suffered more from failure to anticipate ethical decisions down the road than from anticipation.

The other is that some of the more dramatic proposals highlight the ethical issues that are involved more clearly than do the everyday decisions. This means, incidentally, that I will have in mind positive eugenics more than negative eugenics because the former poses more serious problems.

## THE NATURE OF CURRENT CONTROVERSIES

This subject involves sharp controversies. But it is not genuinely a battle between scientists (particularly biologists and geneticists) and humanists (ethicists, theologians or what you will). Rather, among scientists, as among any other group of people, there is a great variety of ethical judgments.

For example, some scientists strongly oppose or caution against the experimental enthusiasm of other scientists. Just three years ago at the annual meeting of the AAAS, Dr. James Shapiro, a member of the Harvard University team that first isolated a gene, dramatically renounced his scientific career, arguing that "so long as men like Nixon and Agnew determine the uses of scientific achievements", scientists should stop producing results that politicians will misuse.

Earlier, Catherine Roberts, a microbiologist, gave up her scientific research saying that we are not now "sufficiently human" to "direct our future by scientifically controlled breeding" and that when we are sufficiently human, "we will have no need for positive eugenics".[1]

Much more moderately, Marshall Nirenberg, a Nobel Laureate has said: "When man becomes capable of instructing his own cells, he must refrain from doing so until he has sufficient wisdom to use this knowledge for the benefit of mankind".[2]

Leon Kass, a biochemist of the National Research Council, has argued that we lack the human wisdom to turn our technology loose on human nature.[3]

And just over a year ago at the International Symposium of the Joseph P. Kennedy, Jr., Foundation, James Watson, another Nobel Laureate, urged Robert Edwards to stop some kinds of medical experimentation on the genesis of human life. And Edwards responded that he would not stop.

Still more recently, an editorial in the *Journal of the American Medical Association* has advocated a moratorium on certain genetic experiments until there is more discussion of the issues at stake.[4]

On the other hand, the late Herman Muller was an outspoken advocate of scientific genetics, and many another scientist has entered the plea for genetic endeavor based either on scientific breeding or on technical methods of modifying germ plasm. **Numerous researchers without much verbalizing are going ahead with work aimed at fertilization *in vitro*, at cloning, or other forms of genetic experimentation.**

We might ask, "Why?" Theodore Roszak has answered in an interesting way. I will quote him. "Consider the strange compulsion our biologists have to synthesize life in a test tube — and the seriousness with which this project is undertaken. Every dumb beast of the earth knows without thinking once about it how to create life: it does so by seeking the delight where it shines most brightly". Why, we may ask, try to do it differently?

The motives, so far as they are stated, are I think, a desire to improve the quality of human life, the sheer joy of experimentation, or the confidence that knowledge and power are inherently good.

I have tried to make the point that there is controversy within the scientific community on these issues. If we look at the community of scholars in ethics, we will find the same controversy, with, for example, Joseph Fletcher enthusiastically endorsing efforts in this direction and Paul Ramsey advocating some strict moral constraints. The argument is not between two disciplines: it is within each discipline.

Now, the differences between the enthusiasts and the critics of genetic experimentation are I think, in a rather small part scientific, involving estimates of the possibilities at stake and the risks involved. I have not the expertise to comment on those scientific judgments. I take the word of somebody who for good or bad reasons has persuaded me.

But to a greater extent, the differences appear to be rooted in ethical assumptions about the morality of human manipulation, the values sought in human existence, and the meaning of human dignity. I want to look at some of those issues.

The claim of the scholar in ethics is not to be more ethical than other people. Ethical scholarship may or may not go with ethical attainment. Prophets, poets, and saints heighten ethical sensitivity. Ethical scholarship investigates the ethical assumptions, arguments, and values that enter human discussion. To the extent that it is historically informed and rationally cogent, it may help people avoid familiar errors of the past and understand their own decisions more clearly.

## FOUR PERTINENT ETHICAL CONSIDERATIONS

Ethical analysis may delineate several issues that frequently emerge in arguments about genetics but are rarely clarified. I here mention four of these.

1. There is something about human selfhood — call it dignity or stubbornness — that resists manipulation. The trouble is that although manipulation is a dirty word, its meaning is far from precise. We might construct a spectrum of possibilities.

Toward one end would be the possibility, apparently real, of implanting electrodes in an organism so as to stimulate pleasure, with the result that the person (if he can be called that) would be continuously titillated into a kind of stupid, passive, silly ecstasy. Almost anybody finds that offensive.

Toward the other end would be relieving a headache with aspirin or an abdominal threat to life with an appendectomy. Almost nobody finds that offensive.

I am trying to suggest that "manipulation" does not of itself suggest a moral judgment, but that we need further thinking about those operations that in ethically offensive ways intrude on the personality as a center of self-determination.

2. A paradox of determinism and freedom seems to run through almost all attempts to improve human life. All science, including healing

science, assumes some causal determinism: do thus and so, and certain consequences can be expected. The same science assumes some freedom on the part of the agent who chooses to initiate causal processes for the sake of desirable goals. The paradox appears in psychological behaviorism as well as in genetic practice; the difference is that the results of genetic alteration may be more radical and more irrevocable. If the would-be benefactor of mankind, whether a preacher or a geneticist is simply carrying out the coded instructions of his own genetic constitution, with no capacity for making judgments that in any sense transcend his own programming, there is something ludicrous in the whole notion that he is intentionally aiming at some good. Yet if persons have something of genuine freedom, there must be circumstances in which such freedom is morally inviolable without the consent of the subject. The principle of consent runs into difficulty, since the unborn cannot give his consent to anything, including his own birth. Yet if consent is totally irrelevant, moral breakdown is imminent.

3. Human life both seeks security and accepts risk. The morality of risk may often be judged higher than the morality of security. Yet there is something immoral in the acts of secure experimenters who subject others to radical risk. At this point there is no sure agreement on which risks are morally defensible and which are not. No life is riskless.

It can be argued that humane interference with natural selection means a deterioration of the gene pool that subjects increasing numbers of the yet unborn to grave risks.

It can also be argued that a callous experimentalism subjects people to risks that degrade humanity. To take a hypothetical possibility that is not seriously proposed, an experimenter might, without moral qualms, subject plant seeds to X-rays or nuclear radiation in order to increase the number of mutations, either in the name of science or in the hope that one-percent of the mutations would be desirable and the rest could be thrown out. The experimenter would not morally do that to human beings. At some point, which I am not prepared to identify precisely, there must be moral restraint about risk, especially subjecting future persons to risk without their consent.

4. Societal good and individual good, although certainly interdependent and to some extent harmonious, do in fact sometimes conflict. Every culture seeks such harmony as it can find between individual and society and settles for some trade-offs. Genetic planning will require some balancing of goods and evils.

However, the problem is more complex than "balance" implies. As John Fletcher has suggested, society does not have very good methods of setting its goals. Those who decide societal goals are actually the powerful members of society, and they tend to decide for their own advantage. Even when they are most idealistic, they project their partisan ideals. There is a curious absolutism in society's pretensions. The theologian who is often accused of being an absolutist in a pragmatic and pluralistic world is actually more apt to be a relativist, questioning the absolutism of power blocs and elites.

The criteria of genetic good set up by persons and societies are culturally conditioned and far from certain. Particular societies or powerful cliques within them claim for their peculiar prejudices the status of norms for all human life for all time.

The record of the present generation of mankind is not so impressive as to convince me that it should become the guardian and director of the human genetic future. Genetic planning, if it were to be highly effective, might well perpetuate certain racial or cultural sterotypes so as to force humanity into a cul-de-sac of obsolescence. The needed balancing of societal and individual goods cannot progress very far until mankind finds better ways of representing societal goods.

Herman Kahn, of all people, has actually proposed — I am not quite sure how far his tongue is in his cheek — that we should have "an index of forbidden knowledge" in which he would include a good deal of genetic knowledge. Thus he says, "Genetic engineering has in it the makings of a totalitarianism the like of which this world has never seen".[5]

Herman Kahn is not a geneticist. Theodosius Dobzhansky, who is, has asked the question: "Are we to have, in place of Plato's philosopher-king, a geneticist king?"[6]

I suppose I fear equally the tyranny of majorities and the tyranny of elites. Scientific elites, no less than ecclesiastical elites or political elites, have sometimes thought themselves immune to the temptations that beset ordinary mortals. The now notorious experiments with syphilis in Tuskegee, although they certainly do not discredit the whole of medical research, suggest that no profession is immune to the temptations of power.

I have defined four issues and have suggested that in each case there is a conflict of values that we need to think through with all the insight and seriousness we can muster. For the sake of the fun of the panel, I might have wished to be more flamboyant or dogmatic, coming down on one side of the conflict of values. I can't honestly do that because I think both sides have real claims upon us and both have real dangers.

It is the destiny of modern man to live with enhanced power resulting from scientific achievement. He will be wise to resist the notion that anything that can be done *ought* to be done. Even so, radical renunciation of power is improbable, and it can be as irresponsible as the lust for power. Learning to live with unprecedented power is probably the most difficult of the tasks that contemporary man has set for himself.

# References

1.  ROBERTS, C. *The Scientific Conscience.*, New York, George Braziller, 1967, p. 23.

2.  NIRENBERG, M., "Will Society Be Prepared?" as quoted by Anderson, W. French, Genetic Therapy. In *The New Genetics and The Future of Man*, (Michael Hamilton, Ed.) Grand Rapids, Williams B. Eerdmans Publishing Co., 1972, p. 120.

3.  KASS, L. New beginnings in life, In *The New Genetics and Future of Man*, *op. cit.*, p. 61.

4.  Editorial: Genetic engineering in man: ethical considerations. *J.A.M.A. 220*:721, 1972.

5.  KAHN, H. As interviewed in the *Times Magazine*, June 20, 1971, pg. 24.

6.  DOBZHANSKY, T. Changing man., *Science 155:*411, 1967.

# IMPACT ON SOCIETY: DISCUSSION

**Rev. Van Wely:** I suggest that we postpone answers for our panel until all the questions have been voiced.

**Mr. Drayton:** I am Bill Drayton, an economist lawyer from New York, McKinsey & Co. Dr. Shinn you have stated very clearly the problem of how to use power which is being developed. What mechanisms would be most appropriate for exercising that power?

One could think of a range from the clear market mechanisms of flooding money and letting individual choice decide, to a mixed mechanism making some mandatory interventions. Or maybe a case by case system using fixed criteria to decide. What mechanism do you suggest?

**Dr. Gliedman:** I am John Gliedman, a writer and psychologist from New Haven. My question concerns the tacit sanguine judgments about history which are implied by the kinds of problem issues involving genetics and society that you have singled out today. I should like to know how, in weighing risks of misuse, you can ignore the lesson of the last fifty years in which one major industrial power — Germany — has had a psychotic breakdown, Japan was captured by militarists, Italy was fascist for a generation, and Russia was ruled by a dictator who almost certainly was insane during his last years. And what do you make of present day countries like South Africa, Greece, and South Vietnam — not to mention post-Stalinist Russia, where, as the Medvedev affair shows, it is apparently considered quite proper to use psychiatry as a weapon of political repression.

**Dr. Raveche:** I am Harold J. Raveche, Statistical Physics Section, National Bureau of Standards, Washington, D.C. Dr. Fletcher, during your talk, you stated that the application of genetic knowledge to man must be kept within the framework of the ultimate goal of medicine — to heal the sick individual or family of disease. The question is, should the goal be extended to include prevention as well as healing? Isn't prevention just as legitimate in the treatment of genetic disease as it is in any other type of disease?

**High School Student:** I am a high school student in Maryland. I have an analogy followed by a more or less rhetorical question. If it were to be established experimentally that I could go out on a bridge over traffic and drop bricks on cars and have a one in four chance of causing some kind of an accident, I am sure if I tried it, I would be hauled away and put in jail. It seems to me that the same type of conditions apply to parents who know that they have some type of harmful genetic mutation who go ahead and have kids. It seems to me the danger to their possible children is just as great as the danger to the drivers on that particular road. And I think that their act would be just as unjustifiable as my dropping bricks in traffic. And I was wondering how you would react to that.

A Scholar: I have a question for Dr. Fletcher. How can you view a future generation as a real entity complete with vested interests and as a party in the debate?

Mr. Lyon: I am John Lyon from the University of Notre Dame. Dr. Shinn, what sense does it make to speak of "future persons"? The conjoining of "future" with "persons" is something that does some violence to logical language.

Dr. Hardin: I don't want to pre-empt what some of the others are going to say about questions really addressed to them. I think the only question thrown my way was by the high school student from Maryland which I thought was rather nice, dropping the bricks off the bridge. It is a very good analogy.

Suppose two parents, both of whom have been identified as being carriers of sickle cell, insist on having children and then when a sickle cell anemic child turns up they turn it over to the State, saying (in effect): "Well, we have socialized medicine, so let the community take care of it".

Note that this is a decision in which the State, the people in general, have had no part. Instead, there is a unilateral power of parents to inflict whatever damage they are capable of on the State. The unconsulted State has to pick up the bills. Is this the price of personal freedom? (Remember, each of us is part of the State). So stated, the issue of freedom to breed is but a special example of what I have previously identified as "The Tragedy of the commons".*

If parents have the unrestricted power to breed, then by gosh, they should have to pay the bills, too. They should not have the power knowingly to produce defective children, knowing in advance what the odds are. If they don't pay the bills, why should they have the power?

Dr. Fletcher: I will pick up where Dr. Hardin left off.

_____

*Hardin, G. The tragedy of the commons, *Science* 162: 1243-1248, 1961.—Eds.

I think there is a big difference between a policeman coming to stop your hand from dropping bricks and putting you in jail for it and the equivalent of what would have to be done to you to stop you from having defective children. Right now, the cost of forcible prevention of child-bearing is a lot steeper than putting you in prison for dropping bricks.

But to try to answer the question directly, I don't like the analogy because the two actions are quite different. In either case, there is harm done. Just to speak personally, from the time I was born, I was taught that to drop bricks was very harmful. I am just beginning to learn fairly late in life something about genetics.

I have had a fairly good education. I was conditioned in my younger life not only to want babies but to think that that was the right thing to do. And I have begun to inhibit myself, a little late, from having babies.

It is quite a thing to recondition a whole generation to the extent that Garrett Hardin recommends. Possibly behind the young man's question was a completely different attitude about child-bearing. How can you turn a whole society around on questions like this? It is very, very difficult to do because when you get at a person's concept of himself as a parent or having children, you get at very deep-seated beliefs. That is as clear as I can be about that question.

Concerning the question of the validity of preventive approach in medical genetics. I would approve of the application of genetic knowledge to the prevention of disease because that is relevant to therapy. I understand the technical problems ahead in preventing the appearance of genetic disease are considerable and the steps between now and preventing, let us say, diabetes genetically are very expensive and problematic, but I would include prevention of disease in therapy.

The question about the future generations is a very good question. Yes, I do consider that future persons have a vested interest in this debate because for the first time in our history we have a more conscious relationship to their possibility of being than we did before. That is our relationship to them, imagining them, the them that we carry in our own genes is more real than ever before. In other words, we do have a responsibility for imagining their stake and the consequences of our genetic decisions to extend the future generations. Therefore, I do in my own cogitations imagine what kinds of consequences or what acts of aggression — I put it as baldly as I can — might we perpetrate against future generations by the decisions that we make now.

**Mr. Lyon:** My name is John Lyon. What bothers me is that linguistic problems or problems of meaning emerge whenever the future is brought into play. Arguments that involve the future, when conjoined with "rights" which pertain to persons living in a "present", seem to make little sense. Something "real", such as a "person", exists only in an *actual* present, and not a conditional future.

**Dr. Hardin:** May I put in just a small word here. I am not sure how many of you know this, but there is an organization in California that defends the "rights" of the unconceived. Stop and think about this. They say, in effect, that every sperm has a right to reach an egg and fertilize it and every egg has a right to be fertilized. Fantastic!

**Dr. Schelling:** I was interested in the question about how we might control the authorities that intervene. It is worth noting that this discussion would have been very unlikely here ten years ago. What has happened in ten years has a little to do with the science of genetics and mainly to do with the legal status of abortion. We are mostly talking about the use of abortion for medical genetics.

We are talking about whether the state should intervene and make mandatory the diagnosis of fetuses and their abortion when indicated, or make mandatory only the screening with suggestions for abortion, whether it is wise to abort fetuses that have been diagnosed in a particular way, and whether abortion should be permitted.

I mention this because it is hard to know which side you are on when you worry about what the government will do.

Garrett Hardin and I were on a television program in which the audience appeared afraid the government would intervene and make mandatory certain kinds of abortions. It is only a very few years ago the government intervened and prohibited abortion.

On many things like the sickle cell trait that was mentioned, the ability of parents to diagnose and abort permits them to avert both a risk and a cost. That is to say, ordinarily they would either run the risk of having a defective child or go without children. If now a probability of one in four or even one in two of a defective child merely subjects them to the risk that they will go 12 weeks pregnant and have to start over, there is an enormous liberation from fear and a widening of choice.

The question still arises, under what circumstances should the government make abortion mandatory? Let me suggest one among dozens of complications. One possibly good use of mandatory abortion is in relieving parents of the painful need to decide for themselves — to allow them to fall back on some higher authority in connection with an action that is not yet altogether socially accepted and to which they may not have been appropriately conditioned in advance. Many parents understand very well how helpful it can be to be able to rely on the excuse, "But that is the way it is supposed to be. That is the rule. That is the law."

It may help, for example, in explaining to a grandparent or to a potential sibling what one has done, to be able to say that as a matter of public policy this choice was not ours to make. And there are many, many gradations between "mandatory" such that it is a criminal offense not to comply and "mandatory" in the sense that you have no financial recourse in the event of an expensive mistake. It is hard to know in many of these cases whether the government is intervening to give you moral support or is intervening in conflict with your interest.

In the matter we are talking about today, it is hard to predict on which side federal agencies, state agencies, local agencies, churches, pressure groups will take a stand. The question is far more complicated than who will control the controllers or how to prevent totalitarian intervention. These are exceedingly complicated problems. Sometimes what appears to be a restrictive rule is moral support; other times, what appears to be a grant of freedom is only the freedom to go and suffer in private the conflicts that can exist between husband and wife, between parent and child.

We are on the threshold of a host of policy issues opened up by the prospect of what used to be called "therapeutic abortion," but now becomes something much more like "optional child-bearing after diagnosis." I don't think there is any easy way even to identify which side various pressure groups, interest groups, and governmental authorities are going to be on.

**A Nurse:** I am a registered nurse. It appears to me that up until this time, you can't see the forest for the trees. It is still the old race and war issues. Would it not be a good solution to marry within your own race and settle the matter?

**Dr. Shinn:** I was asked specifically what sense it makes to speak of "future persons". I have no problem at all in mingling knowledge and imagination because most of the scientists I know tell me there is so much imagination in our advanced scientific thought these days that that would not deter me.

Speaking of future persons seems to me a very common sense sort of thing to do. I believe, given the present state of knowledge, that we would normally regard it as immoral for a pregnant woman to take the drug thalidomide because of what it would do to a future person. So I don't really see a problem there.

The other question that was addressed to me twice had to do with implementation of the issues that I discussed. That is the topic of the next panel, but I think I must say a word about it.

I see this as the problem that has bugged the human race perennially. The first serious genetic proposals I know anything about were in Plato's Republic. They were based on a very primitive science. But the idea was that an elite could plan for people better than they could plan for themselves.

I distrust elites more than Plato did. I also distrust blind anti-intellectuals. I think the main problem of social living is finding that mix of authority that you are willing to assign to government, to various other institutions, and to the individual. This is really a tough problem.

The example of dropping the bricks on the highway is, I think, an interesting one. At the moment I am less concerned with dropping bricks on highways than dropping bombs on Hanoi. I don't know just what device we are going to use on that. I don't know how a society that has not learned how to stop doing that sort of thing is equipped to tell every human mother whether she may or may not go ahead with a child.

I do not mean to say that you have always got to solve your worst problems before you give any attention to others. But as Bentley Glass told us this morning, most of us carry three or four deleterious genes. Although I would have a real problem of conscience about imposing some of my deleterious genes on a future generation, there are many which I do not worry about. I just don't think we are yet at the point of any sound thinking that gives us the right to forbid people to do that.

I prefer to go as far as possible with the educational and voluntary methods, granting the possibility that we may decide that some things are too horrible to inflict. I don't want to close that door dogmatically, but that is presently far down pike. We should be thinking about it, but I am not ready for any such decisions by government.

# IV. HOW CAN SOCIETY'S DECISION-MAKING INSTITUTIONS BE MADE TO FACE THE LONG-TERM CONSEQUENCES OF INDIVIDUAL GENETIC CHOICES?

# SOCIETAL MECHANISMS TO COPE WITH THE NEW GENETICS

**Robert E. Cooke, M.D.**

*Visiting Professor - Department of Preventive and Social Medicine, Harvard Interfaculty Program in Medical Ethics; Vice Chancellor for Health Sciences, University of Wisconsin, Madison, Wisconsin*

## Matters of Fact versus Matters of Morality

*Ought* society to end prenatal life for any cause? *Ought* scientists to develop and apply cloning techniques to human reproduction? *Ought* society to sterilize or otherwise prohibit the reproduction of those who are genetically at high risk? The essential questions facing society concerning the application of new genetic knowledge and technology are not scientific but moral.

To put these questions in an even clearer perspective we might phrase them, "Does the Good Society support, regulate, or prohibit such scientific or technical actions?" For example, *in vitro* fertilization and implantation is a non-moral scientific technique. The risk in terms of subsequent congenital defects is also a non-moral scientific fact. However, the questions "Is the procedure worth the risk?" and "Ought the procedure to be done?" are moral not scientific questions, and must be decided on moral, not scientific grounds.

To use an example from the past, thalidomide was an excellent sedative — it was effective and caused no hangover. Thalidomide also turned out to be an excellent teratogen. Both of these statements are objective, scientific statements. The decision that thalidomide should not be used is a moral judgment based upon the principle that non-injury is a basic obligation of physicians.

## Making Decisions: The Utilitarian Approach

Even if we recognize these questions as moral questions, there still remains a special place for the scientist or professional. How much of a role the scientist ought to play depends on how we view moral decisions and on what moral principles the decisions are to be made.

According to many people, including many scientists, such moral questions must be judged on the basis of their non-moral consequences alone.[1] Their views are utilitarian. They ask, "What are the benefits to society or to the individual now or later from a given moral decision? What is the benefit-to-cost ratio of a decision? What answer to a moral question gives the most happiness or shows the most love?" For example, utilitarians justify sterilization of the mentally retarded by assessing the "practical" effects now or later on society in general.

Similarly, many people consider prenatal diagnosis and abortion for defect to be morally right if the greatest good for the greatest number results.

In utilitarian terms, a question can be asked, "What are the effects of this policy or such policies on future health, future happiness, and future social, psychological and economic well-being?" Many feel that the best judge of practical, non-moral consequences is the professional. He can quantify and measure. He can learn the risks of *in vitro* fertilization. He knows the risks of thalidomide when given on each day of gestation. The scientist or the professional, it is said, is best able to determine the benefit-to-cost ratio of a given policy. If we pursue this line (although I do not agree that the sole criterion is utility), then which professionals are to make decisions? The answer rests with the types of consequences involved and whether we are primarily concerned with immediate or long-range utility.

Yet how should we weigh immediate or long-range utility? How heavily should we consider the possible irreversible effects of our decisions? In what directions do we look for the consequences? How do we avoid the tragedy of embarking on a policy which has unsuspected and possibly irreversible consequences such as pollution?

## Decision-Making by Professionals

In general the geneticist is most to be trusted regarding future *biological* consequences since he has manifested a real concern for the long-term future. The average clinician — pediatrician, obstetrician, internist, radiologist — has shown little concern for the irreversibility of his actions, especially in the use of X-ray or teratogenic or mutagenic drugs. Despite multiple warnings, the use of diagnostic X-ray increases at an alarming rate and diagnostic overkill is now almost routine. But it is worth remembering that the present guidelines for supervision and regulation of clinical experimentation were generated primarily by professionals themselves and that clinicians are in the forefront of those demanding study of ethical issues. Biomedical experts in the field of transplantation have usually been careful and painstaking in deciding policy.

Scientists have imposed self or peer regulation with considerable integrity. But the failures in self regulation, when they have occurred, have been ethically monstrous and seriously damaging to the trust of the community toward the medical researcher. The placebo trials in the treatment of syphilis and in the control of pregnancy are two notorious examples recently brought to light.

Despite a generally good track record, who could expect even the well-informed biologist to measure the behavioral consequences of genetic engineering, such as its effect on child-rearing practices?

At least in the determination of consequences, the scientist is subject to review by his peers. His published work is scrutinized, repeated and confirmed or denied. The professional, on the other hand, as described so clearly by Eliot Freidson in *Professional Dominance*[2], is not subject to significant peer review and is accorded special privileges by law through licensure, even though he may not be qualified to judge consequences in his own field.

So decision-making by the professional or by the scientist working alone is suspect.

### Decision-Making by the Laity

Let us look at the opposite end of the spectrum — decision by non-professionals alone. Serious difficulties certainly arise since many non-moral consequences can only be determined by scientists. One example of such problems is the determination of public priorities by legislators. The legislative process frequently becomes an unreasonable tug-of-war among various pressure groups. Cancer and heart disease are pursued at the expense of probably more critical research areas because of public appeal. The demand for more X-rays as part of routine health care, for more drugs even though potentially harmful, suggests that non-professionals alone are poor judges of non-moral consequences. The average person is abysmally ignorant of the simplest genetic principles or even the simplest concepts of probabilities and ratios.[3]

Thus, it would seem fair to conclude that, if moral decisions about genetics and man are to be made by society on a utilitarian basis, more than one person, more than one group — professional and lay — must participate.

## The Scientist's Role in Moral Decision-Making

If we take a different approach and focus on the *moral* questions alluded to above, if we go beyond the question "What is the scientific risk?" and ask "Should we take the risk?", the decision-making process still should involve scientists. Most human decisions are based only in part on practical consequences. Other moral principles come into play. Some of them are: promise-keeping — the basis of trust; gratitude — in part the basis of dedication and study; justice — both distributive, to each according to his need, and compensatory, making up for past wrongs; non-injury — no harm; self-improvement; honesty; and so on.[4]

Even though such moral principles are not the private territory of the scientist, he must play a role in the making of moral policy since the scientist has pursued the moral obligations of truth and promise-keeping in research as avidly as any group in our society. As Neibuhr[5] has pointed out, science is ordered by a commitment to true and universal knowledge, to conscientiousness in self-criticsm and self-improvement, to faithfulness in truthtelling.

## The Ideal Observer

### A. *Mechanisms for decision-making*

From my earlier statements it should be clear that others besides the biomedical expert must participate in the decision-making process — the psychologist, the clergyman, the lawyer, the sociologist, the layman. But where does this stop? Which layman? Which cleric? On what grounds? On whose intuition?

The following answer may seem overly simplified but to my mind Roderick Firth[6] has supplied as practical an answer as one can find in his *ideal observer* theory. Firth attempts to provide an appropriate and complete procedure for validating moral decisions by specifying the attributes of an ideal moral judge.

The ideal observer would be *omniscient* — know all the facts; *omnipercipient* — imagine vividly how all others would be affected by the decision; *disinterested* — not judge from the standpoint of a particular or vested interest; *dispassionate* — would not make the judgment from the standpoint of an emotional bias; and finally would be relatively *normal* — i.e., not out on the "lunatic fringe".

In other words, the ideal decision demands the following conditions — as far as possible all the facts should be available; all points of view and perspectives should be known and represented; conflicts of interest, even though remote, should be resolved; biases should be minimized, and the answers should make a certain amount of common sense.

Given this brief analysis it seems quite clear that no one person, no one profession, no single group of professionals or laity can possibly meet these criteria. In practice no ideal observer, single or group, is possible, but these requirements provide guidelines for the selection process and for the process of operation after the selection.

The professionals in such a system have the heavy responsibility to provide the facts — all the facts, not simply those that suit their own biases and interests. In this way an approximation to omniscience is attained.

To approximate omnipercipience, the various relevant perspectives must be fully represented. If policy decisions are to be made concerning blacks, then blacks must be involved in depth — not just by token representation; likewise, patients or experimental subjects must participate when decisions concern them. Where immaturity prevents such participation, proper advocacy must be substituted.


B. *Maximizing impartiality: ensuring stable and just conflict resolution*

In the decision-making process each person or group must consciously try to maximize his own impartiality. Do I have an interest — covert or overt — in the outcome? What do I stand to gain? These are questions each member of the decision-making team should ask himself.

Since impartiality of the professional or non-professional may be extraordinarily difficult when strong commitment exists, it is highly likely that disinterest and dispassion may have to be attained by a neutralization of interest and biases by multiple representation. Nevertheless, each participant, although expressing how such decisions might affect him or his constituency, should decide in as impartial a manner as possible. Such is the philosophy of representative government in the legislative branch at least — subject to error, but far more desirable than a monolithic approach.

Precedents for such an approach obviously exist in law but are rare in medicine.

I do not mean to imply that we should substitute a chaotic system of participatory democracy in every local decision with genetic implications. Responsibility for others and respect for the rights of others are absolutely essential for the researcher or clinician; and his dedication to his work or his patients should not be blunted by the removal of responsibility through the imposition of governing, modulating rules and regulations, boards and councils. However, in the formulation of governmental policies, in the creation of legislation, in the development of clinical programs, decision-making groups approximating the ideal observer as closely as possible are essential and represent the best *modus operandi* for all such situations.

### C. *Understanding and communication: key to acceptance of the ideal observer concept.*

Whether scientists and professionals will accept such an approach will depend largely upon the clarity of exposition of the questions being asked. The laity, scientists from other disciplines, the clergy are not being asked to pass on matters appropriate for experts such as the accuracy of enzymatic analyses of cultured amniotic fluid cells. They are being asked to judge whether a severely defective infant is a human being with rights to be respected. Will justice be applied according to his need? Will the principle of non-injury apply? These are moral questions and professionals and non-professionals must communicate if answers are to be found.

### The Basis of Differences Amongst Persons of Goodwill

With such a reasonable approach it seems unreasonable to expect major disputes. Yet, we hear vastly differing opinions from people of good will.

Ralph Potter[7] has shown rather clearly that differences hinge on four variables:

1.  empirical definition of the situation — adequate facts

2.  theological assumptions — religious beliefs

3.  modes of ethical reasoning — largely confined now to utilitarianism or formalism, consequences alone or consequences plus other basic principles to which I have alluded

4.  loyalties — defending one's own territory

If the facts are made available, if the commonalities of religion are appreciated, if common moral beliefs are identified, if loyalties are recognized, if the elements of the ideal observer are approximated, then true communication and decision-making can be achieved.

## Why Concentrate on Principles?

You may well ask, why concentrate on principles? Why not spell out specifics? My reason is this: guidelines, commissions, presidential or legislative task forces or committees or councils are useless, meaningless gestures unless basic moral principles are truly acknowledged and accepted in depth. No easy solutions exist to moral dilemmas!

First, there must be evidence in government of morality — a true dedication to the moral principles of truth, promise-keeping, non-injury, justice — not for white middle class Americans alone but all people everywhere. For example, a civil rights commission means nothing if there is no executive morality. Chaos is mounting regarding sickle cell research because it is seen as a token gesture rather than a moral commitment. A President's Commission on Mental Retardation means *everything* when there is a moral conviction for justice and benevolence.

Where there is evidence of morality, a Federal commission to analyze the moral aspects of research, and even more importantly, application of research can provide significant guidelines to granting agencies. The makeup and the operation of such a commission should follow the general principles I have outlined. Rather than establish rigid prohibitions formed from atomistic approaches, such a commission should encourage analysis of programs by each agency in terms of moral principles. Through this process a critical approach to the ethical issues in each research or service venture would result. Such a commission should define questions, not make rules.

## Preparations Needed for Moral Decision-Making

The Federal establishment should also encourage moral education (as well as genetic education) in the public schools — not religious as such but oriented toward concepts of love and injustice as Lawrence Kohlberg[8] has indicated over the last several years. In this way the general public could learn to understand, appreciate, and in general accept the moral reasoning underlying government policy and avoid the suspicion of an ethical elitism.

The private foundations in this country should encourage universities and medical teaching centers to develop study groups concerned with ethical analysis to promote improved deliberation at the local level, at the bedside, and in the laboratory, as the Joseph P. Kennedy, Jr., Foundation has done at Harvard and Georgetown.

The individual might come to perceive and believe in the *reciprocal relationship* between rights and responsibility, to recognize that with greater education and greater power he must surrender rights and take on greater responsibility — a view of justice as *fairness* described by Rawls.[9]

Local institutions in turn should accept responsibility for moral behavior and not be content, as at present, with a policy of hands-off — adopting the view that what the institution's administration does not know, and what the public does not know, will not hurt them. For example, hospitals are commonly unwilling to establish an ethics committee to encourage discussion of problems of living and dying — even though actions against artificial prolongation of life by unusual means are not unheard of in hospitals. In at least one highly respected institution all such efforts have been interrupted by a policy that the hospital could not establish an official committee that might concern itself with decisions other than supporting life at all cost. The law might prosecute. The public might not understand. What was not known, what was done secretly was institutionally right! A *sub rosa* ethic!

If institutional moral policy can be raised to that of most of the institution's individual members by active efforts of its leaders, then what I have outlined could spark a moral renaissance. At least it might increase our sensitivity to the value of human life.*

*Supported by National Endowment for the Humanities — Joseph P. Kennedy, Jr., Foundation.

# Bibliography

1.  Frankena, William K.: *Ethics*, Englewood Cliffs, N.J., Prentice-Hall, 1963.

2.  Freidson, Eliot: *Professional Dominance*. New York, Atherton Press, 1970.

3.  Leonard, C. O., Chase, G. A., and Childs, B.: Genetic counseling, a consumer's view. *New Engl. J. Med. 287:* 433, 1972.

4.  Ross, W. D.: *The Right and the Good*. Oxford. Clarendon Press, 1930.

5.  Neibuhr, H. R.: *The Responsible Self*. New York, Harper & Row, 1963.

6.  Firth, Roderick: Ethical absolution and the ideal observer. *Phil & Phenom. Res., 12:* 317, 1952.

7.  Potter, Ralph B.: *War and Moral Discourse*. Richmond, Va., John Knox Press, 1971.

8.  Kohlberg, Lawrence: In Beck, C. M.; Crittenden, B. S.; and Sullivan, E. (Eds.) *Moral Education, Interdisciplinary Approaches*. Toronto, U. of Toronto Press, 1971.

9.  Rawls, John: *A Theory of Justice*. Cambridge, Mass., Harvard University Press, 1971.

# THE REGULATION OF GENETIC ENGINEERING

**Stephen Breyer and Richard Zeckhauser, Ph.D.**

*Professor of Law and Professor of Political Economy, Harvard University, Cambridge, Mass.*

*Despite the important social implications of genetic research, proposals for government control, guided by cost-benefit analysis, are ill-advised. Continued public discussion and informal regulation by the medical-scientific community are at present more appropriate.*

Genetic engineering has moved off the science fiction shelf and into the laboratory. Though still in its infancy, it is increasingly proposed as an area for government intervention. What measures of this sort are appropriate?

A cave man asked to speak about the regulation of the wheel, or a Victorian requested to devise a regulatory scheme for electricity, would have no more difficulty than will we in writing of the regulation of genetic engineering. It is not simply that "genetic engineering" itself comprises a nearly limitless range of only dimly foreseen possibilities but also that forms of regulation are as multifarious as varieties of rose.

The government can forbid an activity directly (though this may not prevent it from taking place). Less absolutely, the government can encourage or discourage certain activities through taxes or subsidies. Liquor, tobacco, and perhaps empty beer bottles suffer levies that not only raise revenues but control behavior. Positive governmental incentives are provided for charities, education and diggers for oil. Private institutional control mechanisms take on different form: the free market, the ethics committee of a local hospital, and the approval or censure of one's professional colleagues.

Which of these techniques ought we to rely upon to regulate the development, or the use, of which genetic discoveries? This analysis presents four general, controversial propositions, which it is hoped will help us begin to think about the properties of a proper answer.

1. *Neither theories of technology assessment nor public finance theory will provide much help in deciding whether, how, or how much money should be spent on genetic research.* Technology assessment has recently

been described as "a special type of policy assessment. [It] encompasses the first three steps of the policy making process . . .: (1) identifying possible outcomes . . .: (2) estimating the . . . probability of each . . .: and (3) estimating the utility or disutility of each of the outcomes to the interested parties. . . . It generates data for the decision maker, who carries out the fourth step . . . .: (4) weighing the [expected] utilities and disutilities to the interested parties and deciding among the policy alternatives".[1] This is, in effect, the public finance approach to research funding decisions. Roughly speaking, it consists of an effort to determine the possible outcomes of each research project, value the outcomes, compare the costs of achieving them, and fund accordingly.

Problems inherent in many applications of public finance theory are unusually severe, however, when applied to the funding of genetic research. For one thing, it will prove extraordinarily difficult to predict outcomes accurately. The number of possible outcomes is enormous while the in- dividual probabilities that genetic research will lead to disastrous or utopian results are small. When small probabilities are at stake, dramatic misestimates are likely. Could one have estimated accurately in 1945 — or even yesterday — the probability that nuclear research will lead to destruction of the planet?

Even if we could predict precisely the effect of research on an in- dividual, we would not be helped much if the whole society is involved on some interactive basis. Thus social harm may result when many individuals each employ a genetic technique that each considers personally beneficial. Each family may want a more intelligent child, but it is not obvious what would happen if everyone's intelligence rose by 25%. It is obviously a good idea for some people to adopt children. But what would happen if all families adopted their children? Suppose some people choose to use "ar- tificial reproduction measures." Suppose that all do. A crucial characteristic of these situations is that what one person does affects the welfare of the others. Since individuals' choices in the delicate area of social engineering may not be subject to control, prediction of the social benefit or harm that will result from a genetic innovation is made all the more complicated.

Even if the outcome could be identified, the problem of valuing it would be unusually severe. First, we may encounter changes in tastes. We cannot easily measure the future value of genetic engineering in terms of its utility to a future generation if that generation's tastes or values are, in significant part, the result of genetic engineering. We may not wish to give up the automobile, but, perhaps were we, with our present knowledge, Edwardians, we would choose not to invent it. Nor would we choose to take a drug that would make us prefer turnips to steak, though, after taking it, we would not want to reverse the process.

Second, it is not clear to what extent the existing government has a duty, or a right, to take into account injuries or benefits to future generations, over and above the present desire of the average man to do so. Is there not, for example, a *moral* duty to avoid serious harm to the gene pool — harm that may not reveal itself for, say, ten generations? Alternatively, to what extent ought we to risk defective babies now in order to create a better future?

Third, certain potential consequences of genetic engineering are of a sort that cannot be valued within any cost-benefit matrix. For example, does human creativity, our sense of dignity, our response to human suffering depend to some extent upon a feeling of individual uniqueness? Will such treasured values diminish if men believe they are not random genetically but manifest a consciously determined genetic pattern? Alternatively, does our sense of security derive in part from the fact that loving nurture of parents is coupled ordinarily with genetic identity? To what extent will experiments that require abortion to eliminate mistakes deplete our belief in the sacredness of human life? Would genetic mass production, even with an extensive product line, do the same? Scientific investigation cannot be expected to yield the answers to these questions. But even if it could, we would have no calculus with which to weigh the outcomes that would be identified.

Fourth, it is difficult to take into account the interests of all whom genetic engineering might affect. Even in the simplest case, where parents retain decision-making authority over the process of birth, it is the unrepresented fetus or infant who bears the major risk of error. On the positive side, if genetic research prevents a deformation, it is hard to value the gains to the beneficiary.

Fifth, if there are to be fruits of genetic research, we must know how they will be distributed. Physical integrity is not a traditional economic good. Many citizens would be unhappy if it were to be wholly distributed on a market basis, particularly if the quantities available for purchase were significant. A world in which only the rich could purchase the avoidance of genetic abnormality might be worse than a world in which no one could.

We suspect that research funding decisions will be determined in part by differing intuitive reactions to these problems on the part of many, different individual decision makers. We despair of the possibility of developing a comprehensive decision-making framework that (with a few exceptions) could command near unanimity among funders as to which research projects are desirable and which are not.

2. *Governmental prohibition of genetic research is not likely to be practical or desirable.* Genetic engineering will not descend upon us in a rush but is more likely to insinuate its way into our midst bit by bit. Fundamental life science research has such practical objectives as the diagnosis and cure of inherited diseases, the treatment of infertility, and improved care for prematurely born infants. Even such a frightful sounding experiment as the fusion of the cells of a mosquito with those of a human being is more likely to produce a cure for cancer than to create a flying "mosquito man". Many such projects will offer apparently tangible benefits while their possible harms will appear far more speculative. This makes it unlikely that those who would ban, or severely restrict, such research (even if they comprise the more far-seeing among us) could generate the political force, or will, necessary to do so — particularly if such research also holds out long range promise of, for example, healthier or brighter children. Moreover, such restrictive regulation would not be easy to enforce. Much research is done abroad, and, where research is licensed by a government, much is done in secret. The AEC was able to control atomic research through its monopoly over radioactive material. A monopoly over human eggs would be harder to achieve. At best we could slow the rate of genetic advance; we could not halt the march completely. At the same time, to restrict research severely impinges directly upon other strongly held principles. In science, the relation between experiment and free thought is familial. Although the pursuit of knowledge is not the *summum bonum,* but only one good among many, one hesitates to impede it or to set a precedent that might be used to inhibit other socially controversial research. Indeed, the specter of government law enforcers in the research laboratory, university, or hospital is not to be taken lightly. The advocate of strict governmental control carries a heavy burden of persuasion.

3. *Federal agency type regulation provides at best a very imperfect mechanism for controlling the potential harms inherent in genetic engineering.* Political pressure to allow the use of a genetic discovery that benefits individuals, while risking social harm, can simply sweep aside

agency restrictions and the agency itself in its wake. An agency is no more likely to be able to resist the pressure to allow use of an IQ raising discovery than underdeveloped countries have been able to resist the automobile, even though the widespread use of either may prove socially harmful. Harms that are relatively easy to control — such as the creation of an army of "clones" or mosquito men — may not be realistic threats. Men have had the ability to change the race through selective breeding for many years, and yet have steered clear of this treacherous area without regulatory constraint.

More importantly, the view that an "agency" of wise men or experts can determine the social interest and then enforce its decision is naive. Agencies have proved inept at regulating in areas where values conflict, particularly if they lack precise Congressional instruction. One need only think of the FCC's efforts (or lacks thereof) to control children's television — which may, after all, have a far more pernicious social effect than most foreseeable genetic discoveries. Regulatory agencies also have difficulty in tailoring rules finely to take account of factual differences in roughly similar situations. The Federal Power Commission, for example, has proved unable to set economically proper utility rates. In fact, its well meaning regulatory efforts, when coupled with its need for broad administrable rules, have been partially responsible for a serious natural gas shortage. Indeed, we cannot be certain whether FDA rules, designed to keep ineffective drugs off the market, have, on balance, helped or hurt the consumer. Agency decisions reflect a host of political, administrative, and legal considerations, including not only the reasoned views of experts, but also the interests of agency "clients" and those of its bureaucracy. Agency regulation, of course, may still prove necessary. But if so, some decisions, reflecting the dynamics of small group decision-making, will prove irrational. Some rules will seem insensitive to the need for special case expectations, and some actions will reflect an excessive eagerness to carry out the mandate the agency was given.

There is also the concern that the regulatory process might force to the surface certain issues and decisions that are better submerged. Myths about the ways we conduct our lives can be most comforting. We believe that it is the physician's role to preserve life. Yet we are subliminally aware of situations where doctors have allowed "monster infants" to die. Such a practice is extraordinarily dangerous. It places unwarranted and unwanted ethical and medical responsibility in the hands of the doctor and entails risks of unjustified harm. But how would we want things different? Would we be better off asking a legislature to codify a set of standards to govern such situations? Would the result be more fair or rational? Can we not in some individual cases permit ethical decisions to kill, although we would forbid them were they to become elevated into the general consciousness through formulation of a legal principle?

4. *At present, and in the near future, some aspects of genetic research will call for informal, or decentralized, types of regulation.* Many hospitals, for example, now ask lay panels to review proposals to experiment with human beings. While such panels are sometimes criticized as "rubber stamps", they can at least bring researchers to reveal the scope, details and possible outcome of their work. "Sunlight," as Justice Brandeis reminded us, "is said to be the best of disinfectants." The lay committee can also make the researcher and the hospital aware of nonmedical reaction to their work, forcing them to take account of ethical and social considerations they might otherwise miss. And, continued national discussion of genetic research — its medical and social aspects — can help to evolve standards which will influence experimenters and inform the judgments of lay committees. Professor Freund, suggests that the "voluntary association," not the "criminal sanction," is the proper legal lens for viewing relations among patient, doctor, hospital, and perhaps the community, in the experimental environment. When the subject is genetic research, some or all of these parties must consider themselves trustees for future generations as well.

The experience in the related field of heart transplantation is instructive. Dr. Barnard's initial success fostered a rash of operations around the world. Many of these seemed unwarranted in retrospect. Without any global regulatory procedure, a desirable feedback process operated swiftly. Moratoria on heart transplantation were soon imposed in a wide variety of institutions. The transplant procedure was quickly converted to an experimental process conducted only at a few outstanding research facilities. The lesson is straightforward. In the absence of regulation undesirable practices will spring up. But there exist strong natural forces that tend to contain and reverse them.

To point to the existence of alternative regulatory models is not to deny the need for more direct governmental intervention to deal with certain aspects, or problems, of life science research. Experimentation with human beings, for example, is a topic currently undergoing scrutiny in both the medical and legal communities. Legal safeguards, such as those designed to assure voluntariness, deemed applicable in the general case will apply to genetic experiments as well.

Moreover, genetic and other life science techniques used must be safe for the patient. While the "safety" problem is one that arises with most new drugs, and new medical techniques, one must be particularly sensitive to the risk of injury to the fetus, which cannot look after itself.

Finally, the government must pay particular attention to how life science techniques, such as amniocentesis and genetic counseling, are distributed in society. One might claim that the distribution problem is no different here than when kidney machines, or other life-saving techniques, are at issue. But, the popular, if irrational, association of genetics with fears of a "master race," or — to use an overworked word — "genocide," may make the need to distribute the benefits of such research evenly across all of society particularly pressing.

At this time, the outline of genetic engineering problems can be seen only dimly, if at all. Proposals to institute formal regulatory procedures in this area, for example to license or forbid varieties of genetic research, must be viewed with suspicion. On the other hand it would surely seem appropriate for the federal government to stimulate increased study of, discussion of, and concern about the problems of social and genetic engineering. But this would seem to be the present extent of prudent limits for governmental control.

## Reference

1. FOLK, H. The role of technology assessment in public policy. In *Technology and Man's Future*, A.H. Teich, Ed. St. Martin, N.Y., 1972, pp. 246-47.

# JUDICIAL ROLES IN GENETIC DECISION MAKING

### Daniel M. Singer, Esq.

*Attorney, Fried, Frank, Harris, Shriver & Kampelman,*
*Washington, D.C.*

Decisions concerning human procreation — whether to have children and if so how many, when and of what type — have historically had both public and private components. By and large, private decision-making has been paramount. Attempts at regulation have been ineffective, reflecting both major ignorance and an unwillingness to allocate the public resources necessary to do the job properly.

## NEW KNOWLEDGE SHIFTS THE BORDERS
## BETWEEN PRIVATE FREEDOM AND PUBLIC CONTROL

We can, however, predict with certainty an increase in knowledge which will make possible much more discrete public and individual control over procreation. The public and private temptations to use this newfound knowledge will be many and varied. In some instances, the temptation will be irresistible and the outcome applauded as for example, in the dissemination of birth control information and devices at public expense and abortion on demand. In other instances, the applause may be limited as with regard to compulsory sterilization or mandatory abortion.

But most instances lie somewhere between those considered benevolent and those considered malevolent. In such gray areas public or quasi-public agencies may choose to intervene, believing sincerely that their actions are benevolent and in the service of important social values. Affected individuals may assert that the agencies are ignoring or overriding more fundamental or important social values.

## THE JUDICIAL MECHANISM FOR RESOLVING
## PUBLIC-PRIVATE CONTROVERSY

These conflicts, while exquisitely ethical and moral in nature, are not properly viewed as necessarily struggles between good and evil alone. More properly, these conflicts may reflect different hierarchies of the same or similar values arising out of the common experiences and historical perspectives of the persons involved. There must be a mechanism for resolving these conflicts in a framework that all parties find acceptable.

The judicial system is one possible resolution mechanism which may be useful and necessary in assisting society and its components — individuals, groups, public agencies — to cope with the consequences of new genetic knowledge. Furthermore, the participation of courts may be inevitable in our society since the public policy issues of individual freedom, privacy, and public good are so closely intertwined, especially as judicial institutions already are familiar, reasonably well understood, and enjoy a high level of public confidence.

## TYPES OF JUDICIAL INVOLVEMENT

With new laws making genetic screening mandatory and the prospect of wide-ranging public and quasi-public compulsion to acquire and use genetic data, it is inevitable that the judicial system will be invoked to survey the boundaries between the legally tolerable and the legally intolerable.

Courts will also be invited to resolve the ambiguities that inhere in virtually all regulatory legislation and to protect individuals from inevitable egregious judgments of individual regulators.

## EXAMPLES OF JUDICIAL INVOLVEMENT

Courts have been or will shortly be invited to make decisions in areas where new or recent knowledge in genetics will be deemed relevant or critical to the court's decision. For example, to find a person guilty of a crime the court must find him "responsible" for the crime. In a court case the lawyer for a defendant accused of murder sought to introduce the evidence that the defendant had the chromosomal abnormality called XYY which is postulated to be related to increased aggression in animal behavior.* In the few cases in which the issue has been raised, the courts have found the evidence admissible. Thus, the jury or judge hear the evidence and must make a decision as to whether or not the defendant should be held responsible and put into jail, or be held not responsible for his acts and handled or treated in some other fashion. This must be based on their assessment of the state of the scene at trial time.

---

*This association is disputed. For a recent review see E.B. Hook, Behavioral implications of the human XYY genotype, *Science, 179*: 139, 1973—Eds.

Another example in which the courts have already become involved arises from the shift in abortion laws from prohibitive to permissive. We may anticipate a further shift from the permissive to the mandatory under certain legislatively prescribed conditions. Indeed, there has already been one instance, in Maryland, of a court-ordered abortion — mercifully reversed on appeal. In that case, the abortion was ordered performed on a 16 year old girl upon petition of the girl's mother over the girl's objection. The mother did not like the young man involved and would not consent to marriage which both of the minors sought desperately. Although the case seems so bizarre as to be irrelevant, such court-ordered abortions may become less rare as legislatures attempt increasingly to regulate the quality of the population under their aegis.

As a third example the flurry of recent laws compelling sickle cell screening as a condition of admission to public school will involve the judiciary as mediator.* I have already been invited to participate in one such lawsuit in this area. The lawsuit has not yet begun.

Lastly, I would like to propose to you a hypothetical example which comes from subtle legislation not by direct governmental action. The economic cost of genetic disease can be large. At least a portion of that cost is borne by health insurance companies whose myriad plans cover vast numbers of employed persons and their families.

It takes little prescience to postulate that in the near future some insurance company will offer maternity coverage only if husband and wife agree to submit (at the expense of the company) to broad genetic screening. If a pregnancy is at risk, the mother will be required to undergo amniocentesis, again at the expense of the company. If the fetus is affected, it will be aborted at the expense of the company. But if the parents elect to carry the pregnancy to term, the delivery and after care will not be at the expense of the company.

You might wish to ponder the legal and ethical issues here — whether under our constitutional system, in which we value highly free choice and privacy, courts ought to permit health insurance companies to offer such coverage. Someone will surely challenge any such insurance plan.

The judiciary has already played a role in this area and will do so increasingly as both knowledge and attempts to regulate increase. Courts find

---

*At present, the cost-to-benefit ratio of such screening is unclear—Eds.

it difficult to turn away claims of individuals for protection from the on-
slaughts of government. And, once failing to turn away such claimants,
courts must decide for or against protection of the individual. A decision
either way makes policy.

# CONGRESSIONAL INTERESTS IN THE ETHICAL PROBLEMS OF BIOMEDICAL TECHNOLOGY

Herbert N. Jasper

*Legislative Assistant to U.S. Senator Walter F. Mondale. Senate Committee on Labor and Public Welfare, Washington, D.C.*

## THE NEW BIOLOGY — PROMISES AND RISKS

The new biology holds tremendous promise for achieving progress in prediction, treatment, and even elimination of serious genetic problems. Therefore, we may wish to organize society to exploit this progress.

At the same time, we have to recognize that the new biology poses significant risks for society as we know it. The nature of man and his society may be dramatically changed by certain developments in medical technology. An instructive example is giving every couple the choice of sex of its offspring. All indications are that the preponderant choice would be for male offspring.* If we implemented such choices the sexual balance of our society would change with far-reaching implications for the organization of society.

Other possible choices could be offered to parents — some of which were mentioned by Professor Schelling. For example to be able to choose the size or even to choose handedness of one's offspring could have far-reaching social implications.

## PUBLIC INTERVENTION IN BIOMEDICAL TECHNOLOGY

The Congress of the United States is probably not any better informed about the promise and threat of the new biology than the public at large.

To take the Senate, for example, where I work, there are perhaps not more than four or five Senators whose knowledge of the new biology — and its promises and its risks — is greater than that of the average, well-informed layman. In the House, though my knowledge is less complete I suspect there

---

*This preference is documented but its effect on population composition was held to be temporary in a recent study by Westoff and Rindfuss, *Science 184*:633, 1974—Eds.

are no more. When it comes to staff aides, interestingly enough, knowledge is even more meager because staff on Capitol Hill turn over rather fast. The "institutional memory" in the Congress, as we call it sometimes in Washington, resides with the public official rather than the staff, whereas in the executive branch, where I worked until four years ago, the opposite is true. The staff "go on forever" and the political appointees come and go.

So in the Congress there is a very thin base of knowledge and very limited resources for solving these problems in an intelligent and thoughtful fashion. And that is a danger that we all must recognize. Congress does know that history gives us no reason for confidence that technology will be used only for good. Nazi Germany certainly reminds us that medical technology can be used for ill as well as for good. It wouldn't take very much to persuade members of Congress that medical technology presents serious threats today.

Even if one doesn't take too seriously the risk of intentional damage by scientists, there is the problem of significant harm to society, and to individuals, by accident or miscalculation. An excellent example dramatized by Dr. Robert Cooke is the overuse of x-ray in medical diagnosis. There is also the recent recognition that, perhaps, the standards of protection promulgated by the Atomic Energy Commission have proved to be less safe than was generally thought.

Scientists are not immune from selfish interest. They are not immune from mistakes in judgment. They are not immune from miscalculations.

Recently, we learned about an experiment with "the pill" in Texas, where women were exposed to conception by not being informed that it was a placebo they were taking instead of birth control pills. And some, indeed, did conceive while they thought they were being given contraceptives. There is also the Tuskegee experiment, where the subjects were intentionally not treated for syphilis. We had an experience not too long ago in the Air Force where airmen with strep throats were deliberately not given penicillin, which exposed them to a significant risk of rheumatic fever. Psycho-surgery is on the upswing again and there are clear evidences of excesses of medical practitioners in that field.

While I agree with Dr. Cooke that in general self-regulation is adequate, I also agree that where it has failed occasionally it has failed very badly. Where there is such failure, over-reaction by the public and by Congress could express itself in very undesirable legislation.

There are, of course, ample precedents for public regulation of research and medical practice, as discussed by Professors Breyer and Zeckhauser. The public, if it is stimulated, aroused, or frightened can act decisively through legislation. For example in sickle cell screening, legislation has recently been adopted very widely with some quite undesirable consequences. Programs have been enacted that did not appear carefully thought through, properly adapted to the exact nature of the risk, or sensitive to the possible responses and actions of those detected and informed. As a result repressive measures have been taken against individuals who were found to carry the trait or the disease — which bear no rational relationship to the risks for them, their employers or society. Another example is the thorough regulation of drug therapy by the federal establishment with much clamorous controversy. Persons claim both undue restriction and inadequate safeguards pertain in pharmaco-regulation.

As you can see we have the very clear possibility both for constructive action and for unwise action. What the scientific community has to do is to help establish a framework for public policy-making which both satisfies the public that proper and careful attention is being given to these problems and provides ways to develop optimal regulatory mechanisms, if, indeed, those are necessary.

The challenge is to develop an approach that adequately assesses both the promises and the risks and helps to determine what new structures or procedures are needed, if any. We need also a public and professional consensus permitting the development of responsible courses of action.

The alternative is to do nothing and to wait until a calamity occurs in the form of some monstrous development which will be spread all over the front pages of the papers. And within six weeks, there will be enacted the kind of legislation which may stifle progress for a generation.

## SENATOR MONDALE'S PROPOSAL

Senator Mondale has developed a bill to deal with this problem (Senate Joint Resolution 75). It would establish a two-year study commission with 15 members appointed by the President from a broad variety of disciplines. I don't know that this is the only solution. The commission would study the ethical, social and legal implications of advances in biomedical research and technology. It would make full use of relevant studies conducted by other public or private groups. After two years, it would report its findings and conclusions to the President and the Congress. Its final report would include

"such recommendations for action by public and private bodies and individuals as it deems advisable." Although I am somewhat jaundiced about
public advisory commissions generally, I believe this field lends itself
peculiarly well to study by such a commission since we have no consensus at
all in the field at the moment.

The bill that the Senator introduced, initially five years ago — on the
heels of the first heart transplant — languished in the Congress for the first
four years. It was passed by the Senate in December of 1971 and, unfortunately, was not acted on by the House. I feel sure that it will be introduced again and acted on early by the Senate.* In the House the prospect
for action is good.

I hope that the professional community can organize itself to indicate
that some such approach like this one — which is not rash or precipitous,
and not likely to lead to harsh, stringent, or repressive controls — is
probably a good step to take. It would be far better to have a consensus
reached in the scientific community, so that the Congress might readily
create such a forum for further debate along the lines Dr. Cooke suggested,
than to wait until the public becomes alarmed and acts rashly.

*By the time of publication, it had been reintroduced in the 93rd Congress as S.J. Res.
71.—Eds.

# DISCUSSION

**Dr. Walters:** Dr. Cooke, do you have a comment on what Mr. Singer said about insurance policies?

**Dr. Cooke:** I think he probably didn't realize that there are already discriminatory clauses in almost all health insurance payment for congenital defects. So it would be nothing new to introduce prohibitions against payment if abortion was not performed. Thus coercive policies seem likely. Such coercion prevents exercise of free will and therefore prevents moral decisions from being made.

I would like to ask about the judicial approach. How do you avoid the monstrous consequences of judicial error such as the Holmes decision on sterilization of the retarded? "Three generations of imbeciles are enough. The state's interest in the maintenance of the quality of the species *is* superior to any individual's power of pro-creation" (Buck versus Bell, 1927). I mentioned that medicine suffers from professionalism due to lack of peer review. The same problem exists in the law. How does one handle that kind of problem?

**Mr. Singer:** I don't want to suggest the law is somehow error-free. It is not, any more than any other human activity. But the law exquisitely reflects widely shared community values. By and large, judges, who have no special claim on morality, reach common sense conclusions drawing on a broad range of human experience. Courts do manage over time to follow a fairly consistent course of adhering to what some believe to be the highest standards in the society or to those norms that tend to affect conduct in the direction of a good society. The judicial system has within it certain self-correcting mechanisms (as in the case of the court-ordered abortion) which allow for correction frequently and for reaching a result which is by and large acceptable.

**Dr. Ladimer:** I am now working in conflict resolution in the health area. It seems to me there are some really substantial legally acceptable possibilities for achieving private settlement of disputes. Although using the adversary system, as suggested by Mr. Singer, and therefore subject to appeal, they are handled at the behest and under procedures and principles set by the parties involved. This is the arbitration system, although mediation or other forms of fact finding could be used. It uses selected experts chosen or approved by the parties themselves. One may also have a jury system, if one chooses, as part of it. One can include panels which have as their members, not only professionals, experts, consultants and others, but also members of the community.

I think this approach has a good deal of promise. I would appreciate your comments.

**Mr. Singer:** Any dispute settlement mechanism that is acceptable to the parties involved and into which they put themselves voluntarily should be applauded. For all the law can do, it is not going to save time or money. To the extent that, for instance, medical malpractice issues can be put into the context of a private conflict resolution forum, God bless, it should happen.

On the other hand, it is not at all clear to me that that forum is capable of exposing to wide-ranging comment and criticism the very serious ethical choices that are being made or that will necessarily come into question in terms that Bob Cooke and Steve Breyer have raised here. Those forums, because they are essentially private, may not have the mix of judgments required to reach a decision which is ethically acceptable to a large portion of the population.

One of the things that we are worried about is, how do we get decisions to which people will acquiesce other than by brute force?

**Mr. Burmaster:** I am David Burmaster, a student in Cambridge, Massachusetts. We have heard four points of view today on the prospects for control — self-regulation, executive branch action, court action, and legislative action. The international point of view is conspicuously missing. There is some chance in the distant future, perhaps 50 years from now, that cloning will be a signficant international problem. Some people have postulated that we might get into a cloning race. Other techniques we have heard about today may have ramifications in terms of the conflict between two societies or two nations. What kind of international regulation might be possible to prevent a cloning race or the like?

**Professor Breyer:** I am sorry you asked me that. It is a good time to point out I am not a doctor, actually. I am a lawyer. I don't want to appear too qualified. Law professors typically do not hold Ph.D's.

I won't respond directly, but I think your question illustrates a point that I was trying to make.

I have a great fear of the dramatic. I think that to talk about clones is to introduce the dramatic to an area that doesn't strike me as a real problem. It is possible people could have bred selectively over the past 30 years without any of these scientific developments and produced a master race on the one hand and a group of slaves on the other. And they could have produced horrible creatures to be used for replacement of ... you know, your imagination has no limits as to what we could have done already. And yet we haven't.

I can't rule out the possibility of 20,000 Francos. But I suspect that if that comes about, people will do something about it. And if it requires an international treaty, they will have an international treaty.

I have more concern at this stage with people leaping prematurely to regulation that is too rigid because their minds are fixed on the dramatic example rather than what I see as the more important problems, such as distributing the benefits of the genetic research that has already been done throughout society and worrying about the ethics of human experimentation, which is a real problem at the moment.

**Mr. Singer:** I would agree with what Professor Breyer has said. It seems to me the serious problem areas are not those where one fears obviously evil action. I happen to believe there may be some common sense of decency that pervades most of the world. The evidence is not very good for that, but I happen to believe it anyway.

I think that the most serious problems are ethically ambiguous actions, where you can't see down the road, you don't know what or whose interests to honor or to what extent you should step in and say either "no" or "full speed ahead."

I don't think there is any real chance of protecting against obvious evil through formal national or international action. I think there are great opportunities for professional self-regulation in that kind of undertaking, through informal agreements among scientists generally. But I don't think the serious problems are the ethical horrors.

**Professor Breyer:** Let me offer a weak defense. It is that chemical and biological warfare research did continue for many years completely unscathed by the kinds of regulation you think might be forthcoming for this possible technology.

**Dr. Cooke:** I wanted to agree in a sense, I think the way out is literally "way out" because of economic considerations. If anyone in this audience has taken care of a premature baby she will know the expense that is involved in the care of one premature infant. So if you think you are going to have a race of cloned individuals bred in the test tube, you are mistaken. It is just utterly impossible from the point of view of cost.

I would like to emphasize again the point that has been made as to what tragedy really is, namely a conflict between goods, to emphasize Mr. Singer's point. That is the real dilemma, the real tragedy, in the situation of abortion. It is the conflict between a respect for life and the desire to benefit the parent. This is the basic issue.

The conflict of goods is what gets us into all kinds of moral dilemmas. The conflict is the moral dilemma. The conflict is the tragedy of life. It is not a question of good versus evil. It is the conflict of goods that presents the real problems in our society in this particular instance. We need mechanisms to deal with such conflicts.

**Dr. Boohar:** I am Richard Boohar, University of Nebraska. Mr. Breyer, Mr. Singer, and Mr. Jasper have addressed themselves to the many difficulties involved in regulation of application of genetic knowledge. The speed with which problems are resolved is sometimes a function of the optimism or pessimism of the people involved in resolving the problems. I would like to ask what feeling is found among people in the executive, the judicial, and the legislative areas as to the probability that effective, appropriate regulation for application of genetic knowledge can be achieved in time to prevent some kind of serious social disaster?

**Mr. Jasper:** I can start by saying, as I indicated earlier, that I believe the prospects for formation of a study commission are fairly good. And it is my hope that such an approach might obviate the kind of undesirable crash solution that might otherwise occur.

To underline that, I would like to cite just a case or two to show how quickly the Congress can respond, when excesses become apparent. You all may be familiar with the University of Cincinnati experiment in which whole body radiation in very large doses was given to people suffering from terminal cancer. The Defense Department, which financed the study, has denied that the radiation was thought to have any therapeutic value for the patients. It was administered to assess the consequences of heavy doses of whole body radiation such as might be received in a nuclear war. It also appears that the patients were not adequately informed of the risks or benefits.

It was not more than several months after that information came to light that a rider was attached to the Defense procurement bill which requires a far more elaborate informed-consent procedure in the conduct of experiments on human beings. In this case, I believe the Congressional reaction was sound and sensible, but the potential is present for extreme and ill-considered action, especially if the errors exposed are more alarming than in this instance.

Relevations like the Tuskegee syphilis study or the Texas contraceptive experiment could very quickly lead to narrowly-drawn legislation that is designed to prevent a similar case. I think if any really serious threats to society appear imminent, then very quick action will be taken, possibly with undesirable consequences.

**Mr. Singer:** I would like to add one further thought. Probably within the next 18 months, all of the compulsory sickle cell screening will be ended and screening will become voluntary. It is that anticipation of amendment that has forestalled at least some of the lawsuits that would have been brought to challenge it. So that there is hope that either the excessive will be avoided at the outset or that some kind of corrective social mechanism will be found. I have confidence in professional codes within the various disciplines and governmental standard-setting such as the NIH standards for experimentation on human subjects. They really have a prophylactic effect.

**Professor Breyer:** Well, my only comment — I might be taking the thrust of the question unfairly — is that I was arguing against the view that there are biological, social disasters in the offing that require a vast regulatory program for their prevention.

The kind of bill that Senator Mondale has introduced — that Mr. Jasper was talking about — is quite different. It aims not at comprehensive regulation but at an effort to develop informed thinking on the subject. Such thought will lead doctors and experimenters in the field to focus on the issue and will help develop sensible legislative, or lay committee decisions.

**Mr. Jasper:** Indeed, if I might add to that, the Department of Health, Education, and Welfare did not recommend enactment of the Mondale Bill, largely on the grounds that the mere introduction of the bill in 1968 had spawned so much attention and research in the field that the legislation was no longer necessary. This is, of course, a view with which I don't agree.

**Dr. Shakhashiri:** I am Dr. Shakhashiri from the NIH. In the history of the human race, the choice of which sperm meets which ovum has been made in a variety of ways. It has been regulated. The father of a family or the chief of a tribe would choose which boy would marry which girl. Now, we can tell by the microscope that there are fetuses that are deformed. In either situation, mating or matrimony has been regulated, regardless of method of scrutiny (phenotypic or genotypic), by a value system rooted in the religion of the society in question. Our U.S. society is made up of at least six value systems rooted in four religions: Christianity (Protestant, Catholic, and Orthodox), Judaism, Secularism, and Atheism. I think it is crucial in a democracy that we understand and distinguish between these value systems to become more capable of regulating such matters more intelligently.

**Dr. Walter:** As I understand the question or the comment, it suggests that the discussion of underlying value systems is a prerequisite for making decisions about any problem like genetic engineering or application of genetic technology.

**Dr. Cooke:** I had to leave out a part of my comments. So, Dr. Shakhashiri, I am delighted with your comments, and I agree. I think that there is enormous room in teaching all our children for the consideration of moral development. This is an area that has been very seriously neglected in the last generation and had done poorly prior to that time. There are now some approaches which I hope can be applied.

I referred in my paper to some of the approaches that Dr. Kohlberg has taken at Harvard. And it seems to me these are background for the public to begin to think about moral decision-making. Just as the public is poorly informed on genetics, I think it is just as inexperienced with regard to ethical reasoning.

**Dr. Gliedman:** I am John Gliedman, a writer and psychologist from New Haven. I would like to ask Professor Breyer a question. I agree with you that it would certainly be unwise to ignore the less dramatic ways in which genetic engineering may affect our society and other societies. But I find it curious that — along with the rest of today's panelists — you have not seen fit to consider any of the more dramatic ways in which the genetics of the future may be misused, either deliberately or as the unintended consequence of some well-intentioned social policy. Is this because you think that, both singly and collectively, the nations of the world are strong enough and "sane" enough to render such an eventuality — perhaps in warfare, perhaps as an instrument of domestic repression — highly unlikely? But if so — and this is really the question which I asked during the preceding question period and which no one answered — what in the history of the last sixty years makes you so sure?

**Mr. Breyer:** I am not sure at all. I mean, I can't say that that won't happen, and I didn't mean to imply it won't. But I approach the problem with a different perspective. I see the flaws in regulation — which is, after all, my field — rather than from the perspective of one who sees the flaws in science, which is, after all, your field.

And I suggest that if there is a disaster, there is less that we can do about it than you might think. That sounds terrifically pessimistic. If you could tell me what the disaster will be, maybe I can quickly devise a regulatory scheme. But if you can't we will remain uncertain about just what to do.

**Dr. Cooke:** You know, we are facing genetic disaster right now with the excessive use of X-ray. I have made a proposal to have an X-ray record like an immunization record for every child in the United States. Such an action would avoid repetitive unnecessary radiation. Yet there is practically no interest in this proposal.

If you take care of many patients, you see X-ray over-usage that is producing more genetic damage to the population than all the geneticists put together could possibly do with cloning. It is just too expensive to do much cloning. So right now, unfortunately, we are ignoring important genetic knowledge.

**Dr. Gliedman:** Could I have a brief rejoinder? It seems to me odd, Professor Breyer, that your pessimism was not reflected, however indirectly, in your presentation today. For given that pessimism, might not the most important regulatory issue of all involve education? That is, instead of training more biologists and geneticists, perhaps we ought to be pushing the best minds of our generation into politics or law or even some of the social sciences. Of course, this may smack too much of regulating the practice of pure science for most of the panelists, yourself included. But is it not passing strange that during a symposium devoted to genetics and society, no one has even considered — if only to dismiss — the possibility that the likely costs of a mature genetic technology may so far outweigh the likely social goods that the first task of a conference like this one should be to devise ways of regulating the pace and character of genetic research itself? Herman Kahn now argues that some kinds of science are simply too dangerous to pursue given the world's present level of political and social development. Perhaps he is right that we need a kind of scientific index — a list of forbidden (or at least unfundable) areas of research. I don't know. I only wish that some of the panelists had addressed themselves to these questions today.

**Professor Breyer:** But the trouble is we are talking in a vacuum. Genetic research even on clones for all I know would produce a cure for cancer or will destroy the aggressive tendency in human beings; it may make everyone love each other, end all wars. As long as we are talking about very hypothetical possibilities, I don't think we can sit down and draft a regulatory scheme. That is my basic point.

**Mr. Gliedman:** My point is these possibilities aren't imaginary in the sense that before making any other statement, one has to make a decision about what you do about such things. Maybe a cancer cure isn't worth the risk.

**Mr. Eisenstark:** I am Howard Eisenstark of the Genetics Department at Stanford. I would like to know what is being done or planned to inform the public about genetics, such as television commercials or something.

**Mr. Jasper:** I will start off by saying I don't think any plans are being made. I think the public is terribly ill-informed. Indeed, to a surprising, even shocking degree, the medical community is ill-informed about these problems outside of their own specialty.

As Dr. Cooke knows better than anybody else, the treatment of newborn mongoloid infants is subject to egregious error on the part of medical doctors who don't happen to be specialists in that condition. This applies to a great variety of medical problems. The public is even less informed.

A good illustration of that is a front page article in the Washington Post a couple of Sundays ago on mongolism. The Washington Post is widely regarded (outside the present Administration) as one of the best papers in the country. It assigned a reporter to write a story about mongolism to update our knowledge and destroy some of the misinformation.

The article purported to bring people up to date about what we have learned in the past dozen years. Yet I was struck that the effort fell far short of the current state of knowledge in the field and even continued some of the existing myths about mongolism. If that sounds pessimistic, it is and I am.

**Dr. Lipkin:** At this point I must officially end the symposium. We want to give special thanks from the Youth Council to the Yale Task Force on Genetics and Reproduction which is in large part responsible for the quality of the program and to Ronald Williams and William Drayton, Jr. who have made the production logistically possible.

# V. EDITORS' PERSPECTIVE

# CHOOSING OUR CHILDREN'S GENES: ON THE NEED TO LEARN HOW PEOPLE CHOOSE

**Mack Lipkin, Jr., M.D.**

*Assistant Professor, Departments of Medicine and Psychiatry, University of Rochester School of Medicine and Dentistry*

**Peter T. Rowley, M.D.**

*Associate Professor, Departments of Medicine and Pediatrics and Division of Genetics, University of Rochester School of Medicine and Dentistry*

Choosing our children's genes involves major conflicts between the rights and needs of individuals and those of the other individuals called "society". For example, is there a right to know of a genetic defect one may transmit? Is there a right not to know? If one chooses not to know, to what extent should society bear the consequences? If a couple knowingly takes a high risk and loses, producing a seriously ill child, does society have to help with the burden? Is it fair to the child for society not to help? Can the child sue the parents? Can society's attempts at prevention, since they will always be imperfect, add to any genetic handicaps the additional handicaps of stigmatization?

## THE COST-BENEFIT RATIONALES FOR GENETIC DECISIONS

The primary rationales for preventing genetic disease are reducing suffering and decreasing costs to society. Whether to suffer and live is worse than not to live has been debated since Job. Answers differ due to variations in religion, ethics, experience, and outlook. But most agree that a decreased cost to society is good since this may release resources for other goods. Cost-benefit analysis in genetics thus involves comparing imponderables — the reduction of suffering and cost of care versus the expense of screening, alteration of reproductive behavior, abortion and such invasion of privacy and limitation of options as these involve.

It is widely assumed that cost-benefit analysis, where possible, would show that prevention of a specific genetic disease is worthwhile, or could become so with further research. Such analysis, however, may omit the damage done to those among whom prevention is practiced. Examples include the divorce of affected couples following counseling and discrimination against sickle trait individuals following screening. Unknown are the effects on self-image, emotional state, employability, insurability, and social status.

## GENETIC DECISION-MAKING AND BEHAVIOR

In a democratic society individuals are said to act in their own interest as they perceive it. On what information or experience do persons base genetic decisions? To understand a specific decision may mean to be able to predict it, given the background of the family at risk and of the counselor and the character of the counseling session. The preceding authors and discussants have given much reason for concern about genetic decisions leading to stigmatization, unethical intervention or inaction, deterioration of the gene pool, and thwarting of research and curtailment of services due to inadequate funding.

The concern of all in this volume has been with genetic outcomes and the economic and human costs of effecting them. The behavior of individuals making personal or public choices determines genetic outcomes. For this reason, the science of medical genetics, although absorbing, is of little practical value without a science or art of genetics-related behavior. Without understanding individual decision-making and behavior related to genetic issues of the type and variety discussed in this volume, attempts to influence genetic policy may not have the effect we hope for and may have undesired effects.

Behavior in relation to genetic issues has special features which complicate, but make more urgent, understanding why individuals act as they do. Genetic defects are often hard for laymen to comprehend because they involve unfamiliar conceptual frameworks. Even to the comprehending, one's own genome seems fundamental, immutable, even mysterious. Genomic defects share these qualities. Since human genetics is closely coupled to reproductive behavior, a person's attitudes toward sex and parenthood and his or her self-image inevitably are dominant factors in the feelings and fantasies evoked in genetic discussions and in the process of making genetic decisions. The probabilistic nature of genetic knowledge may be mistaken by some as involving predetermination or punishment.

## GENETIC DECISIONS AND THE PHYSICIAN:
## PRIMUM NON NOCERE

As physicians and genetic counselors we especially need an understanding of genetic decision-making. Patients seek our help expecting maximum benefit and minimum harm — or so we like to think. In any event, we strive to be maximally helpful and, first of all, to do no harm. When someone comes for genetic counseling, the first problem is to define what is maximally helpful in the *patient's* terms. This involves competent diagnosis and knowledge of the genetics and probabilities involved. But much more is needed to be helpful including providing necessary information in a form usable by the individual patient in making a decision. The process requires adequate assessment of each patient's psychologic strengths and weaknesses and the time and skill needed to work through the problems created by the information transmitted.

## TRADITIONAL GENETIC COUNSELING

Some traditional genetic counselors define their role as limited to the diagnostic-pedagogic function. Thus, Hall notes that ". . .the role of the genetic counselor has been that of a neutral educator."[1] McKusick summarizes a more comprehensive process thus, "The central loom for one fabric of medical genetics is clinical genetics — the care of patients and families with genetic disorders. Clinical genetics, like other branches of medicine, is concerned with the answers to three questions: (1) What's wrong? (2) What's going to happen? and (3) What can be done about it?"[2]

Bender's suggestion of a right not to know (*vide supra*, page 73) rests on avoiding the psychological distress of knowing. Clearly such distress cannot be assessed or dealt with successfully in a rigid format, in one hour or afternoon, or by a neutral educator. An emphasis on pedagogy, rather than on establishment of a therapeutic relationship, can undermine the counselor's goals.

Similarly the assumption that he who can diagnose genetic disease will best explain it to a patient is contrary to some experience. Is the medical geneticist, however skilled in clinical diagnosis and laboratory investigation, the most effective in transmitting information? Successful information transmission, one major goal of genetic counseling, requires additional features — talents of its own, experience, some technology (use of instructional aids) and feedback to assure learning. These are not necessarily part of the traditional genetic counselor's approach.

Traditional counseling on the neutral educator model also potentially neglects psychological factors and may be determined more by the needs and values of the counselor than those of counselee. The extent and importance of the prevalence of such problems should be studied. For just as it is unethical to use a new treatment without evaluating its worth and harm,[3] so it is unethical to do genetic counseling with inadequate evaluation of its effects. A genetic counselor who attempts less is like a cardiologist giving digitalis without knowing the serum potassium concentration of his patient. His failure to detect a low potassium and, if such exists, to correct it before giving the drug, may do the patient more harm than not giving digitalis at all.

Improvement of genetic counseling, then, must begin with evaluation of the consequences of the counseling we now do. Improvements based on initial evaluation may then be systematically introduced. These changes must be consistent with broadly derived goals and evaluated in turn. Initial evaluation of any professional service ought to focus on effects. A second stage might study the intent of its practitioners, for example, to be helpful, to pursue knowledge, to advance a viewpoint of the practitioner, or to serve a psychological or social need of the practitioner.

## CONSEQUENCES OF GENETIC COUNSELING

As a first approach, we may consider five categories of consequences of genetic counseling:

1.  comprehension

2.  emotional responses

3.  changes in plans and attitudes

4.  changes in behavior

5.  changes in frequency of affected individuals

Possible determinants of each type of consequence are too numerous to detail but include the counselee's expectations, ethnic group, religious beliefs, and socioeconomic background; psychological attributes and prior health experience; the counselor's attitudes and counseling technique; and the illness involved.

A variety of studies which control these factors must be initiated to analyse genetics-related behavior. For example, a study of counseling could simplify the complex of variables by using only one disease which is relatively asymptomatic. Sickle trait is the subject of several studies now in progress. After screening, uniform counseling can be done. Evaluation can then include tests of comprehension, objective and in-depth evaluation of personal responses, assessment of changes in reproductive or mating plans where appropriate and follow-up to see if plans are carried out.

Each type of consequence presents special considerations.

1) *Comprehension:* This is a major goal of counseling, although it is neither necessary nor sufficient for influencing behavior. How often can a counselor assure that the counselee genuinely understands? Does he retain the information or forget? Is forgetting especially likely if the information is distressing? Can the counselee repeat the information and apply the concepts to his own situation?

2) *Emotional responses:* The emotional responses of counselees to a counseling session range from euphoria to anger or despair. The large variety of counseling situations and the variation among persons and their diseases makes difficult generalization about psychological effects. For example, the psychological impact of counseling the already traumatized parents of an afflicted child where the recurrence risk is low may be very different from the intrusive impact on an oblivious person screened in a compulsory program. A 19 year old engaged boy who was a welder and an ex-high school wrestler was found to have small testes. We were asked to evaluate him for the XXY syndrome. How might full disclosure of his intersex chromosome constitution and probable sterility affect his marriage plans and his sexual identity, or his balances of dependence-independence; passivity-activity; masculine-feminine; heterosexuality-homosexuality; agression-submission. In these cases we do not know what will be most helpful to the patient. Especially when such knowledge is lacking the counselor may act in accord with his own needs alone.

There is, in fact, little information about the range of positive and negative response to counseling. The dynamics of the threat to self-image and the ways to anticipate and facilitate the working through of such a threat have not been adequately studied.

3) *Changes in plans and in behavior:* Changes in behavior refers to actions related to the content of genetic counseling. Such actions are a final observable result of counseling. The first behavior effect available for monitoring may be the expression of new attitudes and formulation of plans such as those for contraception, adoption, or the screening of other family

members. Of particular importance is determining why plans are often not carried out.

## FORMULATING GOALS AND STRATEGY

To choose our children's genes, in either the individual or collective sense, requires, first, the formulation of goals and priorities and, second, strategies for reaching them. The studies suggested here may provide some of the information necessary for choice of both goals and strategies.

What mechanisms will evolve for collective goal-setting remains to be seen but some possibilities are discussed in other articles in this volume. The wise choice of goals will involve balancing of costs and benefits and clearly must take into account how individuals make genetic decisions.

Whatever goals are set, the study of genetics-related behavior is also needed to intelligently formulate strategy. Consider five sample questions of strategy that need answers:

1. Who should counsel — physician or layman, geneticist or psychologist? Should the history and interview, diagnosis, psychological evaluation, and counseling be assigned to different individuals?

2. How should counseling be staged? Is it desirable to divide the counseling process into three separate stages, data collection and diagnosis; counseling per se; and a working through and feedback period? Should each stage be separate in time, setting; etc.?

3. When is the best time to screen or counsel? Learning occurs best in a relatively unstressed atmosphere. Yet often genetic counseling information is presented immediately after the patient hears bad news or has fantasies confirmed. Information should be offered when the patient is ready to receive it rather than when the genetic counselor is ready to give it.

4. What is the best way to convey the facts? Information should be communicated in the way the patient can best understand it, not necessarily in the way the counselor is most comfortable giving it.

5. What kinds of reinforcement facilitate genetic understanding? In medical teaching, the assumption is too often made that learning accompanies the mere presentation of information. If the counselee is to retain the new information, he needs practice in its application.

## SUMMARY

We have argued that all levels of debate and planning concerning genetic issues have as a common focus individuals making choices. It follows that knowledge of the factors influencing those choices should inform such debate and planning.

The neutral educator model of counseling may not be the most appropriate to maximally help and minimally harm. We propose that an improved model be derived from study of human factors in counseling. Such a model may have common elements with the enduring attributes of excellent therapists in any service profession.[4] We are not certain what these attributes are but are certain that they are amenable to systematic study. Such study is of the highest priority. If we readily admit we do not know answers to the simple human questions raised by genetic issues we lose only the illusion of power. But if we do not so admit, we lose the opportunity to help and to learn.

# References

1.  HALL, J. The concerns of doctors and patients. In Hilton, B., Callahan, D., Harris, M., Condliffe, P., and Berkley, B. (Eds.). *Ethical Issues in Human Genetics.*, Plenum Press, New York, 1973, p. 23.

2.  McKUSICK, V.A., CLAIRBORNE, R. *Medical Genetics.*, HP Publishing Co., Inc., New York, 1973, p. xvi.

3.  STRAUSS, M.D. The ethics of experimental therapeutics. *New Engl. J. Med. 288*: 1183-1184, 1973.

4.  ENGEL, G.L. Enduring attributes of medicine relevant for the education of the physician. *Annals of Int. Med. 78*: 587-593, 1973.

171

# SUGGESTIONS FOR FURTHER READING

Bergsma, D., ed., Advances in Human Genetics and Their Impact on Society. *Birth Defects Original Article Series* 8, 1972.

Frankel, M.S. *Genetic Technology: Promises and Problems.* Washington, D.C.: The George Washington University, Program of Policy Studies in Science and Technology, Monograph No. 15, March, 1973.

Harris, Maureen, ed., *Early Diagnosis of Human Genetic Defects: Scientific and Ethical Considerations.* Fogarty International Center Proceedings, No. 6, 1972.

Hilton, B., Callahan, D., Harris, M., Condliffe, P., Berkley, B., eds. Ethical Issues in Human Genetics, Plenum Press, New York, 1973.

Sollitto, S. and Veatch, R.M., *Bibliography of Society, Ethics and the Life Sciences*, Hastings Center, Hastings-on-Hudson, New York, 1974.

Sorenson, J.R. *Social and Psychological Aspects of Applied Human Genetics: A Bibliography.* Washington, D.C.: Fogarty International Center (DHEW Publication No. (NIH) 73-412), 1973.

# CONTRIBUTORS

Harvey Bender, Ph.D.
*Professor of Biology, Notre Dame University.*

Benjamin Brackett, D.V.M., Ph.D.
*Associate Research Professor and Managing Director of the Primate Colony, Department of Obstetrics and Gynecology, Division of Reproductive Biology, School of Medicine, and Department of Animal Biology, School of Veterinary Medicine, University of Pennsylvania, Philadelphia, Pennsylvania.*

Stephen Breyer, Esq.
*Professor of Law, Harvard University, Cambridge, Massachusetts.*

Robert E. Cooke, M.D.
*Visiting Professor — Department of Preventive and Social Medicine, Harvard Interfaculty Program in Medical Ethics; Vice Chancellor for Health Sciences, University of Wisconsin, Madison, Wisconsin.*

John Fletcher, Th.D.
*Director, Interfaith Metropolitan Theological Education, Inc., Washington, D. C.*

Garrett Hardin, Ph.D.
*Department of Biological Sciences, University of California, Santa Barbara.*

Y. Edward Hsia, M.R.C.P.
*Associate Professor of Human Genetics and Pediatrics, Yale University School of Medicine; Director, Genetics Clinic, Yale-New Haven Hospital; Member Yale Task Force on Genetics and Reproduction, New Haven, Connecticut.*

Mrs. Hubert H. Humphrey
*Washington, D. C.*

Herbert N. Jasper
*Legislative Assistant to U. S. Senator Walter F. Mondale, Senate Committee on Labor and Public Welfare, Washington, D. C.*

Michael M. Kaback, M.D.
*Associate Professor of Pediatrics and Medicine, Associate Chief, Division of Medical Genetics, Harbor General Hospital, UCLA School of Medicine, Torrance, California.*

Irving Ladimer, S.J.D.
*Adjunct Associate Professor, Mount Sinai School of Medicine, City University of New York; Special Counsel/Health Care, American Arbitration Association, New York, New York.*

Mack Lipkin, Jr., M.D.
*Assistant Professor of Medicine and Psychiatry, University of Rochester School of Medicine and Dentistry, Rochester, New York.*

Leon Rosenberg, M.D.
*Professor and Chairman, Department of Human Genetics, Yale University School of Medicine, New Haven, Connecticut.*

Peter T. Rowley, M.D.
*Associate Professor, Departments of Medicine and Pediatrics and Division of Genetics, University of Rochester School of Medicine and Dentistry, Rochester, New York.*

Thomas C. Schelling, Ph.D.
*Professor of Economics, Harvard University, Cambridge, Massachusetts.*

Roger L. Shinn, Ph.D.
*Union Theological Seminary, New York, New York.*

Daniel M. Singer, Attorney
*Fried, Frank, Harris, Shriver & Kampelman, Washington, D. C.*

James R. Sorenson, Ph.D.
*Associate Professor of Socio-Medical Sciences, Boston University School of Medicine, Boston, Massachusetts.*

Richard Zeckhauser, Ph.D.
*Professor of Political Economy, Harvard University, Cambridge, Massachusetts.*

# DISCUSSANTS

Garland Allen, Ph.D. (Discussion I)

Harvey Bender, Ph.D. (Discussion II)

Bonnie Blustein (Discussion II)

Richard Boohar, Ph.D. (Discussion IV)

Benjamin Brackett, D.V.M., Ph.D. (Discussion I)

Stephen Breyer, Esq. (Discussion IV)

George Brosseau (Discussion II)

David Burmaster (Discussion IV)

Robert E. Cooke, M.D. (Discussion IV)

Ann Desmoyers (Discussion II)

William Drayton, Jr., Esq. (Discussion III)

Howard Eisenstark (Discussions II & IV)

Julian Ferholt, M.D., (Moderator, Discussion II)

John Fletcher, Th. D. (Discussion III)

Mark Frankel (Discussion I)

Bentley Glass, Ph.D. (Discussion II)

John Gleidman, Ph.D. (Discussions III & IV)

Garrett Hardin, Ph.D. (Discussion III)

Y. Edward Hsia, M.D. (Discussion II)

Frances Ivker (Discussion II)

Herbert N. Jasper (Discussion IV)

Evelyn W. Jemison (Discussion II)

Michael M. Kaback, M.D. (Discussion I)

Irving Ladimer, S.J.D. (Discussions I & IV)

John Lyon (Discussion III)

Maurice J. Mahoney, M.D. (Arranger and Moderator, Discussion I)

Harold J. Raveche, Ph.D. (Discussion II)

Leon Rosenberg, M.D. (Discussion II)

Thomas C. Schelling, Ph.D. (Discussion II)

Zekin A. Shakhashiri (Discussion IV)

Roger L. Shinn, Ph.D (Discussion III)

Ruth Silverberg, M.S.W. (Arranger, Discussion II)

David M. Singer (Discussion IV)

James R. Sorenson, Ph.D. (Discussion II)

Richard A. Tropp, L.L.B. (Arranger, Discussion IV)

Richard A. Van Wely, S.T.M., Rev.
      (Moderator and Arranger, Discussion III)

Virginia Walbot, Ph.D. (Discussion I)

Leroy D. Walters (Moderator, Discussion IV)